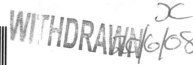

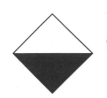

appearance

# Health psychology

Series editors:
Sheila Payne and Sandra Horn

Published titles

# The psychology of appearance

## Nichola Rumsey and Diana Harcourt

**Open University Press**

Open University Press
McGraw-Hill Education
McGraw-Hill House
Shoppenhangers Road
Maidenhead
Berkshire
England
SL6 2QL

email: enquiries@openup.co.uk
world wide web: www.openup.co.uk

and Two Penn Plaza, New York, NY 10121-2289, USA

First Published 2005

A catalogue record of this book is available from the British Library

ISBN-10: 0 335 21276 X (pb)    0 335 21277 8 (hb)
ISBN-13: 978 0335 21276 7 (pb)    978 0335 21277 4 (hb)

Library of Congress Cataloging-in-Publication Data
CIP data has been applied for

Typeset by RefineCatch Ltd, Bungay, Suffolk
Printed in Poland EU by OZGraf. S.A.
www.polskabook.pl

*To Alex and James, who have never made me feel guilty for being a working mum. Big thanks guys. You're the best.   NR*

*To my friends and family who offered the best support just when it was needed.   DH*

# Contents

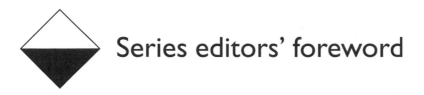 # Series editors' foreword

This series of books in health psychology is designed to support post-graduate and post-qualification studies in psychology, nursing, medicine and paramedical sciences and health psychology units in the undergraduate curriculum. Health psychology has grown, and continues to grow rapidly as a field of study. Concerned as it is with the application of psychological theories and models to the promotion and maintenance of health and the individual and interpersonal aspects of adaptive behaviour in illness and disability, health psychology has a wide remit and a potentially important role to play in the future.

This exciting and most welcome addition to the series has been produced by researchers from the Centre for Appearance Research, at the University of the West of England, in Bristol, United Kingdom, which has established a national and international reputation for research and teaching in the area. The book builds upon the strong research and practice development agenda for the authors who have collaborated with key charities and other funding bodies. Personal appearance as experienced and construed by the self, by others and via cultural norms, is a fundamental issue in health and wellbeing across the lifespan, but has been relatively neglected as a topic of study in the past. Changes to appearance can be caused by genetic anomalies, disease processes or accidents such as burns, which occur at different times over the lifespan. Interest in and concern about outward appearance have a very long history but have a special relevance now, when appearance-related anxiety is widespread and pervasive, affects an increasingly younger age group, and is sometimes associated with potentially life-threatening behaviour. Concern about appearance influences decisions about whether to engage in health behaviour and crucial medical treatment and surgery, and may involve clin-ically unnecessary surgical procedures and the risky misuse of medication. The cosmetics industry markets strongly promises of enhanced appearance. Where there is an obvious visible difference in someone's appearance, the personal and interpersonal challenges associated with being outside the norm bring additional difficult and ongoing challenges. These are all issues of central relevance to health psychology.

In this book, reports of the literature and research findings are enriched by quotes from those affected. The text begins with a history of the significance of appearance-related concerns and goes on to consider the methodological and other challenges facing researchers in the area – including the inadequacy of existing models and theories. The writers then offer a new framework for appearance-related research. Throughout the book, the psychosocial aspects of appearance concerns, for those with and without visible differences, are explored from research findings and personal viewpoints. Current provision of care is examined, and more effective interventions and support mechanisms are proposed. The book ends with a look at challenges for the future and the potential contribution of health psychology to this important area of human experience.

There is much food for thought in this eminently readable book, in which the salient issues are presented with clarity, academic rigour and humanity. Thus, it shows contemporary health psychology at its best.

*Sheila Payne and Sandra Horn*
*Series Editors*

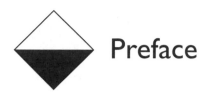 # Preface

The invitation to write this book generated the time-honoured mix of emotions, but despite some trepidation (relating most notably to time pressures and self-doubt), the challenge was irresistible. We knew the book would be timely in view of the growing need to point up the relevance of the role of appearance in areas of key concern to health psychologists, including adjustment and wellbeing, understanding and changing health behaviours and in adherence to treatment regimes.

We experienced the usual problems in making and defending the time necessary to write. As deadlines loomed, we twice escaped the pressures of the daily grind and retreated to an idyllic seaside setting in Cornwall. The combination of stunning scenery and the lack of invasive technology (no fax or Internet connection and only a distant mobile phone mast) provided the perfect environment for writing and gave us the impetus necessary to complete the task.

Appearance is a universal topic with relevance to all. We all have an appearance of some kind, and, with the exception of identical twins, there are more than six billion unique appearances in the world. Our outward appearance plays a part in the minutiae of daily life – from our frequent encounters with others to its role in a broad raft of health behaviours. Although people have always been interested in outward appearances and have actively engaged in a range of activities to manage their looks since records began, in current society appearance concerns have reached epidemic proportions. Ninety-two per cent of teenage girls in the UK are unhappy with their body shape (Wardle, reported in *The Times*, 25 September 2004) and the proportion of teenagers and adults now prepared to engage in activities which carry significant health risks is increasing rapidly. As Linney (2004) pointed out, although it is illegal to discriminate against any person on the grounds of ethnic origin, gender, sexual orientation or marital status, it is still widely accepted that we make stereotypical judgements (especially 'snap' judgements) of people on the basis of their outward appearance. Historically, appearance-related research has been the preserve of social and clinical psychologists, but it is now clear that many aspects are also directly relevant to health psychologists.

Why is appearance so relevant to health and wellbeing? First, people's feelings about their appearance can be an important influence on their decisions about whether or not to engage in health behaviours (for example, the desire to change body shape may be a more powerful motivator to embark on an exercise regime than the wish to reduce the risk of heart disease), yet an explicit acknowledgement of the role of appearance is absent in most models within health psychology. Second, many types of illness and subsequent treatment involve appearance issues (for example decision making about treatment options for breast cancer – see Chapter 6). Third, dissatisfaction with appearance is widespread and increasing numbers of individuals are electing to undergo appearance-altering interventions that have inherent health risks (for example, cosmetic surgery, tattooing). Fourth, appearance issues may affect adherence to treatment regimes (for example, weight gain as a side effect of the treatment of diabetes). The numbers of people with disfiguring conditions is increasing, in part due to advances in medical and surgical techniques which mean that ever larger numbers of people are surviving after disfiguring treatment. Having an appearance that is visibly different from 'the norm' can bring with it a host of challenges that impact on psychological functioning, and which may involve ongoing treatment (see Chapter 4). Finally, as health care professionals deal with increasing numbers of people presenting with appearance concerns, they are looking for research evidence to underpin their work. While recognizing the impact of appearance concerns on their patients, they are unclear how to offer appropriate care and support. Increasingly, they are looking to health and clinical psychologists to advise them in this respect. The topic of appearance is therefore relevant to a wide range of applications in health psychology.

## The structure of this book

We did not set out to offer an exhaustive review of all the research in this area. This would have required several books, and a very protracted retreat to Cornwall. Instead, we set ourselves the task of pulling together the strands in this rapidly expanding area, with an emphasis on those issues of most relevance to health psychology. In places we have included 'voices of experience', particularly those of people affected by a visible difference. We chose to do this partly to illustrate researcher findings, but also because these words are so much more eloquent and thought provoking than those written by people who are not directly affected by the issues explored in this book. We hope those of you who are curious to know more will seek out the texts and readings we recommend at the end of each chapter.

SECTION 1 examines historical, contextual and methodological issues. Chapter 1 is an introduction to the area, tracing the history of the significance of physical appearance through to current 'epidemic' levels of appearance-related concerns. Chapter 2 considers the many challenges facing researchers in this area and offers a new framework for appearance-related research given the inadequacy of existing theories and models in the area.

SECTION 2 examines the psychosocial concerns, needs and difficulties experienced by those troubled by their appearance. It begins with a review of appearance and image issues for those without visible difference (Chapter 3), looking at the difficulties and distress experienced by those affected across the lifespan. Chapter 4 focuses on the psychosocial difficulties experienced by those with visible difference, including a detailed consideration of the specific issues associated with a range of aetiologies including cancer, burns, skin conditions and rheumatoid arthritis. In Chapter 5 we examine the psychological factors that contribute to vulnerability and resilience to appearance concerns, including a variety of cognitive factors, the impact of social support, the role of appearance in self esteem and the importance of social skills.

SECTION 3 examines ways of addressing psychosocial concerns through support and interventions. In Chapter 6 we consider the provision of care as it currently stands for people with or without a visible difference, and we include an overview of the problems of an exclusively biomedical approach. In Chapter 7 we examine the potential for more effective support and intervention including specialist psychosocial support, school-based interventions and the potential role of health promotion campaigns and the media.

Finally in Chapter 8 we look ahead at the challenges for the future, including the dilemmas surrounding technological advances such as the current trend towards ever more flawless computer-generated faces and bodies and the resulting impact on norms of appearance and new health-related technologies including antenatal screening, genetic engineering and facial transplant surgery. We also examine the potential contribution of health psychology research and practice in this area to continuing efforts to change health care delivery to more effectively meet the needs of those experiencing distress from appearance-related difficulties.

## Contributors

The Centre for Appearance Research (CAR) has attracted some excellent researchers and colleagues over the past few years. We are grateful to those who have made valuable contributions to this volume and who have constantly challenged our thinking about the topic. Kate Gleeson is a Clinical Psychology Reader at the University of Bristol, and Hannah Frith is a senior lecturer in Social Psychology in the School of Psychology, University of the West of England, Bristol. Hannah and Kate have a wealth of experience in qualitative research into identity and appearance – and were great writing companions in Cornwall. Alex Clarke is Consultant Clinical Psychologist at the Royal Free Hospital, London. She has enormous expertise of clinical practice in the area of visible difference and has published widely on the topic of interventions and the provision of care in this area. Claire Phillips is a research fellow funded by The Healing Foundation and based in CAR, specializing in research into the psychosocial impact of burn injuries. We would also like to thank other colleagues for their indirect contributions to the book. Emily Lovegrove is a research fellow in the CAR funded by the United States NIH and working on a project researching quality of life in adolescents with craniofacial conditions as part of a consortium headed by Professor Donald Patrick and his team at the University of Washington, Seattle. Anna Fussell is an invaluable member of the team and we would like to thank her for her cheerful help and support during the preparation of this book. Tim Moss and Emma Halliwell are recent additions to CAR. This book was well underway by the time they joined us, but there will be no escape for them should there be another time!

**The language used in this book**

Among those who research and practise in the area of 'disfigurement', much agonizing has taken place concerning the most appropriate language to describe a visible difference. The terminology used to date has a predominantly negative focus (for example, disfigurement, abnormality, deformity, defect and so on). These words derive from the biomedical approach to care and its problem-focused, pathologizing emphasis in treating presenting conditions (see Chapter 6). There is now a groundswell of opinion (see for example, Eiserman 2001; Strauss 2001) that negative terminology is at best unhelpful, and at worst exacerbates the difficulties experienced by those seeking help. Some writers and researchers have striven to compensate for the prevailing negative focus by using terminology such as 'visible distinction' (see Partridge 1999). However, this approach has not met with universal approval among those affected (especially those experiencing particular difficulties), and does not have the advantage of evoking the current shared understanding triggered by the word 'disfigurement'. We have chosen the middle ground and where possible have used terminology that is less negatively framed, but hopefully still widely understood (for example, by replacing 'disfigurement' with 'different' where appropriate). Amanda Bates (a postgraduate researcher at CAR) has helped us do this and we would like to thank her for her invaluable suggestions. In addition, we have chosen to highlight recent research efforts that explore the more positive aspects of being visibly different.

Finally, another member of the CAR, Natty Leitner, recently reviewed, in a personal communication to the authors, the contents of major health psychology journals and concluded that appearance was a highly pertinent, yet usually overlooked aspect of research in health psychology. This is an area which is ripe for the involvement of health psychologists, and we hope that by the time they get to the end of this book, readers will be left in no doubt as to the relevance and importance of studying appearance. We hope that they too will be convinced of the need to put this stimulating and diverse topic higher up the health psychology agenda.

**Further reading**

Throughout this book we have referred to the charitable organizations, Changing Faces and Let's Face It which provide psychological support to people living with a visible difference and to others who are affected. Both organizations have useful and informative websites that include links to other organizations able to offer condition-specific support and we direct readers to these sites for further information: www.changingfaces.org.uk and www.lets-face-it.org.uk.

CHAPTER
1

# Appearance matters: the history of appearance research

*(with contributions from Hannah Frith and Kate Gleeson)*

Evidence for the fascination humans have with physical appearance comes from a rich variety of sources, including mythology and legends, anecdotes from history, fairy tales and a variety of contemporary sources. Examples of the interest we as a species take both in our own appearance and the way we present ourselves to others have been derived from as long as 30,000 years ago, when in Africa people chose to decorate their faces (Bates and Cleese 2001), and from examples of portraiture from 23,000 BC (Kemp et al. 2004).

There is evidence that we have an innate tendency to be fascinated by faces. From a few days after birth, infants gaze at faces in preference to any other stimuli, with the movements of eyes capturing attention (Bruce and Young 1998). In settings when it is unlikely that a gaze will turn into a social encounter, such as sitting in a train carriage, in a waiting room, or perhaps sitting in front of the TV, many of us enjoy the luxury of being able to observe the faces, figures and clothing of others, idly speculating about the links between people's outward appearance and their temperament and occupation.

We are also preoccupied with our own appearance. The first true mirrors were made in 1460 by the Venetians, who worked out how to create clear glass. People enjoyed seeing themselves so much that this quickly turned into big business. The del Gallo brothers found out how to create a perfect reflection in 1507, but the Venetians managed to keep the knowledge to themselves for more than a century, despite the efforts of spies and diplomats from other countries who tried to discover their secret (Bates and Cleese 2001). We examine our own appearance thousands of times in our lives, and most of us respond to the urge to check out our reflection in shop windows or mirrors when the opportunity arises. The sight of our familiar appearance does much to reassure us about our identity; however, we are taken aback when our appearance does not conform to our own internalized self-image – for example when harsh lighting offers a version of ourselves which appears older than our internalized self-view, or when others claim that a photo we consider unflattering is in fact a good likeness. Physical changes to the body, and in particular the face, powerfully affect the way we experience ourselves and take some time to assimilate into our self-view. This phenomenon is recognized by health care professionals who carefully manage the first post-operative glimpse in a mirror following major trauma or surgery. Those affected can be shocked for some time afterwards when catching sight of an unexpected image (Bradbury 1997).

For as long as records have existed, there have been examples of those who have invested in adornment to enhance their appearance to others. For some, the lengths have been considerable; for example, the damaging lead-based skin-whitening paste used in Elizabethan times, the arsenic preparations used in seventeenth-century Italy for the same purpose (Bates and Cleese 2001), saucer-shaped discs inserted into lips among tribes in Brazil and Africa, foot binding in China and neck lengthening in Thailand. Parallels can be drawn with the contemporary use in western societies of the toxin botox to smooth wrinkles, the widespread application of painful and unsightly teeth braces for later cosmetic gain, dietary restrictions or supplements, piercings, tattoos and the willingness of increasing numbers of people to undergo the risks and expense associated with cosmetic surgery. Over the centuries there have been protests about the health risks and also the deception involved in some self-presentation strategies. For example in England during the 1700s, there was an outcry among men in relation to the personal adornment of women. The art of seduction by appearance was considered to be deceitful, as the 'true' face was masked. In 1770 in England, a law was drafted that permitted divorce on the basis of this 'deception'. However, it was apparently unenforceable and was allowed to lapse (Bates and Cleese 2001). More contemporary debates also involve the rights and wrongs of altering appearance through surgery (see Davis 1995).

Whatever our personal beliefs, most of us actively attempt to influence the way we look (for example, through our choice of clothing or hairstyle), either to conform to perceived norms of appearance, or out of a desire to express our individuality (Newell 2000a). However, not all appearance-related changes are under our control. As part of the developmental cycle, the physical body and our perceptions of it go through changes. Some of these may be desired (for example, the changes associated with physical maturation in adolescence are welcomed by many, as is the toning of the body through exercise), while others, such as those resulting from ageing or illness, are less welcome (Newell 2000a). All changes, whether developmental, illness-related or self-induced, take place in the context of a society which both in the past and currently places a heavy emphasis on outward appearance. Gilbert (2002) asserted that for millions of years, the currency of attraction and the imperative of appearing attractive to others has shaped the evolution of minds and brains. We have come to believe that appearing attractive to others is in our own self-interest, as we will have better access to desirable social resources such as friendships, lovers and long-term relationships. Many legends were woven around the influence of outward appearance, with most implying that the possession of beauty is all-important and confers power to the possessor. Lakoff and Scherr (1984) refer to a Greek legend concerning the three powerful goddesses Hera, Pallas Athene and Aphrodite. All three squabbled about who should receive a golden apple inscribed 'For the fairest' which was flung into the middle of a wedding celebration by the goddess of discord, Eris. The wedding was thrown into disarray by their tantrums, and each attempted to bribe the appointed judge. Among the consequences of their efforts to win the prize was a ten-year war. The central tenet of the legend is that to be acknow-ledged as the most beautiful was of paramount importance and to some, at least, worth virtually any cost.

Although we may shrug off legends as imaginative stories lacking relevance to more contemporary beliefs and behaviours, examples of the enduring emphasis on physical appearance over the years abound. Fairy tales and children's stories reinforce pre-existing stereotypes. Sleeping Beauty is cast under a spell by wicked and ugly witches, Snow White's stepmother regularly checks her appearance in the mirror and worries that her beauty will be eclipsed by her stepdaughter; Cinderella's beauty is envied by her ugly stepsisters and generations of children have quaked at the sight of the evil cartoon character Captain Hook. In the 1920s, the strap line for Camay (soap) advertisements was: 'Every woman is in a beauty contest every day of her life'. Haiken (2000) quotes from a newspaper advertisement for plastic surgery published in the USA in 1946: 'To a homely girl, life may seem an endless succession of embarrassments, frustrations and anguish until she decides one day to have a plastic surgery operation'. The extent of our investment in appearance as we begin the twenty-first century is reflected in a beauty industry estimated to be worth a staggering $45 billion worldwide (Bates and Cleese 2001). McGrouther (a British plastic surgeon) recently quoted a statistic that the cost of advertising lipstick alone in the UK was £12 million each year.

The current vogue for speed dating (in which decisions whether or not to proceed with a date are made in the first few minutes of an encounter) leaves no doubt as to the imperative for many of optimizing their physical appearance. Gleeson and Frith (personal communication) have coined the term 'scopic economy' to refer to a contemporary societal economy that relies on being 'scoped' by others, and in which some physical attributes (including slimness, a youthful appearance and symmetrical facial features), are valued more than others. Our position in this economy is negotiable to some extent through interventions such as diet, exercise and surgery, and increasing numbers of people engage in these activities to maintain or improve their status.

Our physical appearance provides powerful cues for identity and recogni-tion by others. This is the first information available to a perceiver, and is continuously on show during social interaction. Whether we like it or not, there is no opting out of this process (Gleeson and Frith, personal communication). Most of the time we do not have a choice about whether or not we engage in encounters with others, or about the fact that others respond to the visual self that we present (Frost et al. 2000). The face is on show more than any other part of the body. It is a hugely sophisticated communication tool and a crucial component in the formation and maintenance of relationships, providing a bewildering variety of important social signals which are detected, interpreted and responded to by others. Hughes (1998) highlighted the importance of the face in daily life by referencing the many verbal expressions which crop up in everyday language, including 'facing up to something', 'two faced' and 'losing face'. Hatfield and Sprecher noted that 'other information may be more meaningful, but is far harder to ferret out' (1986: 72). It is a staggering statistic that there are six billion human faces on the earth at any one time (Bates and Cleese 2001), with every one of them unique as the result of a complex interaction of genes, developmental stage, life experiences and environment. Consequently, faces are used as the unique identifier on passports, identity cards and driving licences. With all this complexity, how do we make judgements of what is beautiful or ugly; attractive or unpleasant? On what basis do we decide who we wish to interact with, and what interaction style would be most appropriate?

## Judgements of beauty and the desirability of being attractive to others – then and now

Bates and Cleese (2001) suggest that the phrase 'beauty is in the eye of the beholder' is a cliché, maintaining that across the world, the judgements made of beauty and the foundations of attraction have much in common. They propose a melting pot of influences including Greek philosophy, evolutionary biology, mathematical formulae (specifically that an inherent pleasure is derived from a symmetry of features which can be specified, as in the ancient Greek notion of The Golden Mean), an innate tendency for humans to favour baby-like features (for example, large eyes and mouth and small nose capitalized upon with great success by Disney), and personal preferences based on past experience.

Darwin was one of the first to discuss the possible universality of facial attractiveness across cultures by noting in 1871 that explorers had remarked to him that indigenous people around the world shared similar standards of beauty. There is some evidence that worldwide in current society, people agree to a large extent on which faces are considered beautiful. In 1993, the anthropologists Jones and Hill (1993) travelled to two relatively isolated tribes in Venezuela and Paraguay. Previously, the tribes people had little contact with people outside their own village. They had no access to TV, and so had not seen images of people from elsewhere in the world. They were shown a range of photos from various cultures and asked to rate them for beauty. The judgements were compared with ratings of the same photos by people from Russia, Brazil and the USA. People in all five countries chose female faces with delicate jaws and chins together with large eyes. Other studies confirm smooth skin, large eyes and plump lips as desirable (Kemp et al. 2004). However, there appears to be more agreement concerning judgements of female faces than those of men and also a consensus that physical features are not the only aspect to contribute to judgements of attractiveness. Lively animated faces are popular, presumably because they indicate a high probability that the person in question is fun to be with. Similarly, a mobile face may be more attractive in real life than one which is more beautiful but lacking in expressiveness. Agreement in judgements of beauty relate predominantly to first impressions. Variation creeps in as relationships become established and other factors affect our judgements of a person.

Despite the high levels of agreement about what comprises beauty in current society, there are examples of changes over time. In men and women, the Greeks and Romans prized eyebrows that met over the middle of the nose. A prominent forehead, aquiline nose and a 'cupid's bow' shaped mouth were favoured. Ancient Egyptian female 'beauties' were portrayed with rounded bodies, a very pronounced chin and a jutting lower jaw. Around 400 years ago (in the 1600s), a double chin was fashionable for both sexes, as the well off could afford to eat well. In Renaissance times the emphasis was on harmonious facial and bodily proportions – Durer and da Vinci favoured the gap between the eyes being equivalent to the width of the nose. In the late nineteenth century, the fashion of corsetry for women emphasized the ideal of the hourglass figure. In the 1950s, a fuller faced and figured woman was more popular than currently. In the 1960s and 1970s, before the widespread recognition of the dangers of skin malignancies, a deeply tanned face was fashionable (once again, an external sign of affluence for those who could afford to travel to sunnier climes). Men grew their hair long, and female models were portrayed as being particularly slim with close cropped hair. In the late 1990s, models were cast with pale skin, appearing unsmiling and frail. Rugged, muscular men were in vogue in the 1970s and 1980s, whereas more boyish, waif-like ones took front stage in the 1990s. In recent decades, an increasing value has been attached to a youthful appearance in many walks of life. An increased emphasis on the desirability of appearing fit and healthy, together with pressures in the employment market have all conspired to denigrate the visible signs of ageing. In response, people are taking ever more drastic steps to counter the signs of advancing years.

## Making judgements of morality and personality from physical features

In addition to providing the material on which judgements of beauty and initial assessments of mutual attraction are made, the notion that character can be read from the face also has a long pedigree. Many great writers have subscribed to this view, including Cicero ('The face is the image of the soul'); Shakespeare ('There's no art to find the mind's construction in the face') and Oscar Wilde ('It is only shallow people who do not judge by appearance'). Aristotle, who is credited with one of the earliest objective studies of the face, concluded among other things that 'men with small foreheads are fickle, whereas if they are round or bulging out, the owners are quick tempered ... The staring eye indicates impudence, the winking, indecision. Large and outstanding ears indicate a tendency to irrelevant talk and chattering' (cited in Burr 1935). In the eighteenth century, a Swiss clergyman, Johann Lavater, wrote a huge treatise on physiognomy. Lavater (1789) considered the nose to be an indicator of taste, sensibility and feeling; lips of mildness and anger, love and hatred; the chin, sensuality; the neck, flexibility and sincerity. He also gave a clear description of an equation between outward appearance and goodness. 'The morally best [are] the most beautiful, the morally worst, the most deformed'. The Victorians considered themselves expert face readers, attributing moral judgements and personality type on the basis of the exterior shape of the head. This was a science with royal patronage. Queen Victoria apparently had her children's heads measured and analysed (MacLachlan 2004) and during the nineteenth century, Camper (cited in Bruce and Young 2001) apparently attempted to measure intellect from the angle of the nose. Galton (1883) developed an interest in the facial appearance of criminals and studied photographs of prison inmates. He described their appearance as 'villainous', stating that 'it is unhappily a fact that fairly distinct types of criminals breeding true to their kind have become established, and are one of the saddest disfigurements of modern civilisation'. He took his work one stage further by developing composites from the photos of criminals, and was allegedly disappointed that the result looked 'surprisingly handsome' (Perrett and Moore 2004). Lombroso (1911, cited in Bruce and Young 1998), a French criminologist, proposed that all mankind was divisible into 'criminal' and 'non-criminal' types. He claimed that the 'born criminal' was characterized by facial asymmetry, a low sloping forehead, prominent brows and anomalous teeth. Lombroso proposed that in order to reduce crime, all the people who looked like criminals should be rounded up. To aid the authorities, he even provided a set of pictures indicative of 'criminal types' (MacLachlan 2004)!

The Second World War Holocaust in Germany was preceded by an orchestrated smear campaign portraying Jews as ugly and evil, which included the widespread publication of cartoons depicting Jewish people as hunched, grasping figures with enormous hooked noses (Lovegrove 2002).

Although many segments of more contemporary society might pride themselves that racial prejudice on the basis of appearance is no longer acceptable, in the lead up to the Rwandan genocide in Africa, the Hutu state radio station broadcasted propaganda describing the Tutsis as morally degenerate and physically impaired (Lovegrove 2002).

From a scientific point of view these theories have been totally discredited; however, folklore linking aspects of appearance to personality has persisted throughout recorded history, and judgements based on the appearance of others are still in common parlance. For some, red hair is taken as a sign of a fiery temper; small eyes are indicative of a lack of trustworthiness. An idle browse in a station bookshop led to the recent discovery of *The Complete Guide to Chinese Face Reading* (Dee 2001). This book describes the art of Kang Xiang, in which the shape of the face, eyes, nose, mouth and ears are a map of our character and life. If a person has a bent or broken nose, a squint, a twisted lip or blemished eyebrow, allegedly there is discord in that person's life. Media moguls also contribute to the perpetuation of myths linking appearance and personality. The physical depiction of characters in Disney cartoons for example, varies markedly depending on whether the characters are 'goodies' (large eyes, symmetrical faces, slim figures) or 'baddies' (heavy facial features and sometimes scarring). Despite evidence to the contrary, we continue to harbour some deep-seated associations between outward appearance and inner character.

Over the years psychologists have attempted to tease out the factors involved in these processes. Secord (1958) gave participants a brief verbal 'personal' account of two imaginary characters. The accounts were the same except for the words 'warmhearted and honest' or 'ruthless and brutal'. Participants gave indications of the appearance they expected the characters to have by rating 32 physical characteristics on seven-point scales. Secord found that 25 out of the 32 characteristics were significantly different as a function of the personality accounts, with participants using 'average' characteristics for the 'warmhearted and honest' person (for example, average width of nose), but unusual features (a very narrow, or very wide nose) for the 'ruthless and brutal' person.

In 1972, Dion and her colleagues also harked back to the days of face reading, in coining the phrase 'what is beautiful is good' to explain their research findings which suggested that people assign more favourable personality traits and personal qualities to people they judge to be attractive. Eagly and colleagues (1991) carried out meta-analyses of findings of research into physical attractiveness and the associated stereotypes. They concluded that the more attractive are perceived as more sociable, socially skilled, to have better mental health, to be more sexually warm and dominant. However, the news is not all good, as attractive people are not seen as having greater concern for others or a better character. Feingold (1992) studied the behavioural correlates of appearance, and reported that the more attractive had better social skills and more same-sex friends. In addition, they reported less loneliness and lower social anxiety. However, no significant relationships were found between physical attractiveness and some other personality characteristics including sociability and levels of psychological wellbeing.

Cook (1939, cited in Bruce and Young 1998) asked people to estimate the intelligence of students from photographs. Respondents' estimates were completely unrelated to the actual IQ or performance scores, but there was a high level of concordance among the estimates made by participants, who considered higher intelligence to be associated with greater symmetry of facial features, a serious expression and a tidy hairstyle! More recent research has been contradictory, and Shepherd (1989) concluded that there were no grounds for thinking we can accurately read intelligence from faces. Eagly and colleagues (1991) pointed out that this may be because physical attractiveness is not strongly linked to intellectual competence in popular culture.

Bull and colleagues (1983) also demonstrated that a considerable degree of agreement exists in our judgements on the basis of facial appearance, despite the fact that these judgements are inaccurate. Participants were shown full-face photographs of Conservative and Labour politicians. The authors found agreement in ratings of political inclination, but that these were not related to actual affiliation. Those judged to be Conservative were rated as being more attractive, more intelligent and of higher social class than the 'Labour' politicians. The judgements made did not vary according to the self-reported political leanings of those making the ratings.

It would appear that although when pressed, we acknowledge that there is much more to an individual than just their physical appearance, we use stereotypes freely and unthinkingly. Our culture's obsession with physical perfection is demonstrated in every magazine, billboard, film and television programme. In this context, we continue to make swift, inaccurate judgements of personality, intelligence and a host of psychological attributes – often agreeing with others about what aspects make faces look more or less appealing.

**Reactions to visible differences**

In parallel with the positive attributions made on the basis of beauty and attractiveness, explanations to account for the occurrence of an unusual appearance have been consistently negative over the years. Shaw (1981) reported the existence of one tablet dating back to 2000 BC, which forecast that the infant 'that had no tongue, the house of the man will be ruined – that has an upper lip overriding the lower, people of the world will rejoice'. Shaw also noted that in classical times, the gods were thought to create 'monstrous' infants, either for their own amusement, or to warn, admonish or threaten mankind. Babies with physical impairments (and sometimes their mothers) were routinely sacrificed in an attempt to placate the gods. In myths and legends handed down over the years, the faces of witches, gargoyles and trolls are depicted with abnormalities or damage. Medusa's punishment for being too beautiful in her mortal life was to make her grotesque through the transformation of her hair into hissing serpents. She was so terrible to behold that others turned to stone if they saw her, and eventually she was killed by her own reflection (MacLachlan 2004).

In the Middle Ages, foetal impairments were thought to be the product of the union of the mother with an animal and it is these beliefs which may have been reflected in mythological images such as the Centaur and the Minotaur. The practice of executing those affected has been recorded as recently as the seventeenth century, and Shaw (1981) recorded that in 1708, Frederick V of Denmark ruled that no person with a facial deformity should show themselves to a pregnant woman. Historically, unusual faces have also been associated with mental health problems. Hogarth's eighteenth-century paintings of depravity and inmates of mental institutions are notorious for portraying unattractive or impaired faces (Munro 1981). Francis Bacon (Bacon, 1597) has been attributed with the statement that 'deformed people are commonly vengeful – returning in coin the evil that nature has visited upon them' (see Newell 2000b). People with severe physical impairments have been recruited to circus freak shows, allowing audiences to indulge in voyeurism (MacLachlan 2004). Although there have been some sensitive screen, literary and media portrayals (for example, John Merrick, in the film the Elephant Man, and the promotion of Falklands veteran Simon Weston – who survived severe burns – as a hero), in the main, visibly different faces and bodies have been linked over the years with evil or monstrous behaviour in films such as *The Phantom of the Opera, Frankenstein, Nightmare on Elm Street*, and as terrifying zombies and werewolves depicted in horror movies. Unfortunately, these more recent examples are not confined to the screen. In Nazi Germany, physically disabled people, those with learning difficulties and people with mental health problems were sent to death camps along with Jews, gypsies and homosexuals.

What are the origins of prejudices that work to the advantage of those considered physically attractive and to the disadvantage of those who are judged to be unattractive or visibly different? Various explanations have been offered including the remnants of instinctive beliefs, the associations generated by the historical infliction of outward signs to indicate a lowly status in society, such as that of a criminal or slave. Lovegrove (2002) noted that in India, hundreds of years BC, noses were cut off as a punishment for adultery), or the processes of social conditioning and reinforcement resulting from, among other factors, media exposure to biased views of what is 'normal' and 'abnormal'.

More recently, the occurrence of physical differences has been attributed to stellar influences, seminal and menstrual causes, or the sighting of 'unlucky' animals during pregnancy (for example, a hare resulting in a cleft lip in the foetus). It would be reasonable to assume that these beliefs have died out, but Shaw (1981) noted that even in recent times among some African tribes, a man with any kind of physical impairment cannot be elevated to chieftaincy. In some rural communities in the Indian sub-continent, families of babies with physical disabilities are stigmatized until prescribed purifying rituals have been performed. Strauss (1985) noted rela-tively recently the occurrence of infanticide and selective malnutrition of children born with physical impairments in contemporary China and Brazil, and Gittings (2001) noted that over 60 per cent of the 100,000 abandoned children and babies in China each year have physical differences. In a survey of 200 women reported in 1981, Shaw solicited explanations for the occurrence of congenital impairments. Although many respondents offered quasi-medical explanations, others attributed the blame to maternal behaviour (for example, the excessive consumption of strawberries or red cabbage during pregnancy resulting in an infant with a port-wine stain), and although these explanations derived from folklore were in the minority, unfavourable preconceptions about the personality of people with facial differences were still common.

In Goffman's essay 'Notes on the Management of a Spoiled Identity' (1963), he explored the area of difference and stigma from a sociological viewpoint. In his writings he combined a number of groups including criminals, people with disfigurements and those set apart from others by their ethnic origins or religious beliefs under the heading of stigmatized people, defining stigma as a situation in which an individual is 'disqualified from full social acceptance'. Goffman was particularly interested in the interactions between members of the general public and a stigmatized per-son. He maintained that when 'normals' (his word) meet such a person, they may be uncomfortable because the stigmatizing feature is unusual. As they lack experience to guide their behaviour they will be anxious not to behave inappropriately, and nervous that the person may be defensive or aggressive as a result of their attribute. They will also be concerned that there will be other, non-visible differences associated with the stigma. Discredited people will also be at risk of displaying unusual behaviour, as they will be anticipating possible rejection by others, and will consider it likely that other aspects of their personality will be linked to their visible difference.

Goffman's insightful thoughts have been developed further in con-temporary research relating to the effects of disfigurement (see Chapter 4). Sambler and Hopkins (1986) originally coined the terms 'felt' stigma (defined as the individual's belief that they are likely to experience negative reactions from others because of their socially undesirable characteristic) and 'enacted' stigma (the explicit rejection or isolation of a person as the result of their difference) based on their work with people with epilepsy. Few of their respondents could actually identify an act of rejection, leading Sambler and Hopkins (1986) to note that a fear of stigmatization can develop even in the absence of actual rejection. Jones and colleagues (1984) provide six dimensions of stigma that influence the degree to which a 'marked' person is stigmatized and which are relevant in the context of a visible difference: concealability; the progression of the condition; disruptiveness to communication with the individual; the aesthetic qualities of the condition; the origin of the condition (the degree of stigma is greater if the person is perceived to be responsible for the condition); and the risks to the person when exposed to the affected other. Clifford maintained that the person who is visibly different 'is marked, not because he fails to achieve the ideal state of being beautiful, but because he has failed to achieve a minimum standard of acceptability' (1973: 6). Trust (1977), who has a large facial birthmark, wrote that the visibility of an unusual facial appearance means 'walking around as a permanently branded second class citizen'.

The instinctual theories focus on the idea that we retain a legacy of behaviour handed down from a time when natural selection shaped the perpetuation of physical and behavioural attributes. The tendency for mothers to allow or cause their offspring to die if they manifest any kind of impairment at birth is present in some animal species. As the preference to look at the visual pattern offered by a normal face is present very soon after birth, an additional component of instinctual rejection may be a degree of confusion or unease when we encounter anything abnormal (Bruce and Young 2001). A facial difference may also 'instinctively' be interpreted as a sign of a more profound internal, cognitive or emotional disorder.

Theories highlighting processes of reinforcement and social conditioning emphasize the pressure within groups to conform to socially defined norms. In current society, appearance-related norms are defined and perpetuated in many ways, with imagery in print, on television and in films offering a particularly powerful point of social comparison through a constant barrage of messages about how we should look and behave (McCabe and Ricciardelli 2003). In addition to the use of physical appearance as part of the stereotyped characterizations in films, TV and magazines, advertisers associate beautiful people with a desirable lifestyle, presenting cultural schemata that appearance and thinness are absolutely vital for success and happiness (Tiggemann 2002). The numerous attractive and flawless faces on the covers of magazines, in films and in advertising provide information which reinforces and shapes our cultural conceptions of beauty, attractiveness and normality. At the same time, the pervasive association of distortions of physical appearance with evil and fear is also evident in stories, books, films, cartoons and comic caricatures. Rumsey (1983) reported stories written about photographs of people with facial disfigurements by a large sample of seven year olds which reflected negative prejudices and stereotypes that were heavily influenced by comic book story lines and popular television programmes. Whether or not the origins of our responses to visible disfigurements are instinctive, the issue of whether the media influences the perpetuation of appearance related stereotypes for the majority of the general population is not in doubt.

Haig-Ferguson (2003) offered a fascinating slant on the pervasive influence of the media and other social norms in people's self-perceptions of appearance through his analysis of interviews with ten blind people. He found that, although the participants were not directly exposed to media images, these and other social and cultural ideals still influenced their self-perceptions through the medium of everyday talk with friends and family:

> You [talk about why] people want to be David Beckham, and the girls want to look like Britney Spears and Christina Aguilera.

> Well, you know that being obese isn't good just by hearing other people . . . you somehow know really by the language used . . . and people would be bullied at school for being fat.

As for sighted people who are able to monitor the responses of others, Haig-Ferguson's participants were very aware of being judged by others on the basis of their appearance, and also responded to the feedback of others about how they looked. Participants wanted to 'look good' both for their own self-esteem and also because they felt they were on show as representatives of other blind people. The author felt that their aims in relation to 'looking good' were more modest than those of some sighted people, focusing in the main on passing as 'normal' and looking smart and tidy. Interestingly, in the same way some sighted people complain of being judged by others on a particular aspect of their appearance that they dislike, several participants felt that their blindness clouded judgements of them by others:

> A big appearance problem for me is being judged on the way I do things because of being blind.

Participants were also able to clearly articulate their body ideals and their concerns about ageing and appearance, though once again, the weight attached to some aspects of their aspirations may be different to that of sighted people. Haig-Ferguson singled out the most salient aspects as being the desire to achieve and maintain a healthy and fully functioning body, rather than concerns about wrinkles and sagging skin.

The stereotypic judgements made by others of people with visible differences can play a large part in the negative experiences reported by those affected. When challenged, many people would acknowledge that happiness and quality of life involve much more than outward appearance – yet most of us also pander to the superficial ideology in which beauty and attractiveness are linked with all things desirable. How have psychologists tried to study and understand these pervasive interpersonal processes?

## The emergence of literature concerning the psychology of appearance

The history of appearance research makes interesting reading, with clear examples of the influence of the societal context on the activities and conclusions of researchers working in the area. As early as 1921, Perrin stated in the *Journal of Experimental Psychology* that 'just why the physical characteristics of individuals should exert so profound an influence over their associates furnishes an interesting topic of speculation'. Holmes and Hatch (1938) took up the challenge in a study in which the facial beauty of students was rated. The authors reported that a greater proportion of the 'beautiful' women (34 per cent) had later married than the merely 'good looking' (28 per cent), 'plain' (16 per cent) and tactfully termed 'homely' (11 per cent). Some pockets of work on self-perceptions of appearance also emerged in the 1940s and 1950s. Secord and Jourard designed the first scales to measure self-ratings of subjective appearance in 1953. However, these isolated forays into this area of research were the exception rather than the rule, and Perrin would have been disappointed that so few researchers felt compelled to take up the challenge until the 1960s!

Some writers (for example, Kleinke 1974) suggested that by avoiding the study of facial appearance, psychologists could refrain from supporting the unpalatable view that looks really are important in how a person is judged. Adams and Crossman made the point that 'from a scientific perspective, little is known about the psychological importance of beauty' (1978: 84) and in 1981 Berscheid talked of a collective reluctance to acknowledge the true impact of physical appearance. Cash and Pruzinsky commenting on the level of expenditure on cosmetic products in western societies, noted that: 'although this practice would seem to be a fascinating aspect of human behaviour on the basis of its generality and resilience, social-behavioural scientists have largely ignored the phenomenon so plainly in front of their eyes' (2002: 8).

It is also interesting to note the comments of Hatfield. In 1966 (at that time publishing under the name of Walster; see Walster et al. 1966), she found that in a study of 752 university students carried out in the context of a dance during Freshers' Week in which partners were randomly chosen by computer, the only predictor of an individual's liking for and desire to subsequently date a potential partner was physical attractiveness. However, Hatfield was discouraged by colleagues from publishing her findings. She later reflected that appearance was almost universally regarded as a frivolous and superficial attribute. Interestingly, in the context of the current boom in cosmetic surgery, she noted that in the 1960s, requests for plastic surgery were assumed to be a symptom of neuroticism, and those requesting surgical intervention were routinely assumed to be at risk for psychopathology. Similarly, the only reasonable justification for dental or orthodontic treatment was an improvement of function, not of aesthetic appearance. However, she reflected that by the late 1980s the climate had changed. Lawyers, judges and juries had become interested in the potential of building legal cases around the detrimental impact of impaired physical appearance on social and economic opportunities and on self-esteem. They were eager for evidence to support their cases and early research findings were largely supportive of their arguments. In addition, Bull and Rumsey (1988) noted that interest in the role of appearance in the process of impression formation was increasing as people had become more geographically mobile and were coming into contact with larger numbers of unknown others for the first time.

Reflecting the increasing overtness of the interest of the general public and psychologists in appearance, the 1970s and 1980s saw a considerable expansion in research activity centred around two main themes – first, studies exploring the kinds of judgements which are made on the basis of physical appearance; and second, the relative effects of various aspects of appearance on these judgements. The majority of the early studies tended to oversimplify the processes involved in appearance-related impression formation and stereotyping. The mood of the time was summed up by Udry and Eckland:

> Everyone knows that it is better to be beautiful than to be ugly. There may be some people who would prefer to be bad than good. Some might even prefer to be poor than rich. But we take it on faith that no one prefers to be ugly. The reason for this must be that people expect good things to come to the beautiful. Folklore tells us that beautiful girls marry handsome princes and live happily ever after. Heroes are handsome and villains are ugly.
>
> (1984: 48)

In parallel, a third literature emerged relating to body image (broadly defined as self-perceptions of appearance). The focus of this research was heavily influenced by the finding that the preponderance of body image concerns related to weight and also by increasing concerns about the escalating incidence of eating disorders.

**Judgements made on the basis of physical appearance**

Most of the research carried out in the 1970s and 1980s claimed pronounced and positive effects played by facial attractiveness in liking, dating and in longer-term relationships, but the majority were methodologically weak and conceptually naïve. Many studies involved undergraduate students rating head and shoulder photographs and almost all lacked ecological validity. In 1981 Berscheid claimed that levels of physical attractiveness had been shown in numerous investigations to be an 'extraordinarily important psychological variable', with pervasive and strong effects resulting in numerous preferential social treatments. In their comprehensive review,

Bull and Rumsey (1988) felt that Berscheid's claim was overstated, arguing that the simplistic conclusions reached by researchers using photographs of people in hypothetical situations were misleading. With hindsight, researchers in the 1970s and 1980s were making their own contribution to the escalating societal hype associating physical attractiveness with all things desirable! Bull and Rumsey summarized this research in 1988 in relation to five main areas. These are reviewed briefly in the sections which follow.

### Attraction: liking, dating and longer-term relationships

Studies in the 1960s and 1970s claimed pronounced effects of facial attractiveness on liking and dating. However, later more realistic studies which included additional variables (for example, attitude similarity) revealed more complex interaction effects. Using evidence derived from ratings of photographs of married couples, Murstein (1972) outlined an 'exchange-market' or 'equity' model. This theory proposed that people would choose others of similar levels of attractiveness to themselves as long-term partners. In relationships where this was not the case, Murstein proposed a compensatory mechanism of wealth, status or prestige. Subsequent evidence for a small to moderate effect for the 'matching hypothesis' was also found in same-sex close friends (Cash and Derlega 1978), and Feingold (1988) reported a significant correspondence in the attractiveness levels of married couples, dating partners and even in close friendships.

### Facial appearance and the criminal justice system

Whether as the result of repeated exposure to media stereotypes or through other mechanisms, many people over the years have believed that a relationship exists between facial appearance and criminality (Linney 2004). Although there is evidence that people do share stereotypical notions of what a criminal appearance is like, the evidence that people who commit crimes do have certain types of facial appearance does not exist. In the 1960s and 1970s, there was a widespread belief that facial differences might contribute to criminal tendencies. This led to plastic surgery being offered to prison inmates to increase the chances of them making a satisfactory adjustment after their release into society. Spira and colleagues (1966) reported that fewer of those who had undergone operations returned to prison (17 per cent) than the non-operated peers (32 per cent), but other later reports concluded that there was little objective evidence that surgery was beneficial.

There are contradictory findings concerning the effects of facial appearance on the attributions of others of responsibility for crimes. Several early studies suggested 'jurors' were more lenient in their judgements of guilt and in the sentencing of defendants with a more attractive facial appearance (Bull and Rumsey 1988). However, most studies were contrived, comprising unrealistic simulations of courtroom scenarios, and the amount of variance explained in more realistic studies was less. In later studies, it was a relief to find that the severity, nature and type of crime, and the amount of detail given concerning both the perpetrator and the victim moderated the impact of appearance on sentencing decisions. In addition, the physical attractiveness or otherwise of the 'defendants' had a greater effect on the judicially inexperienced compared to those with more courtroom experience.

### Facial appearance and the educational system

Research on the effects of facial appearance in the educational system also enjoyed a hey-day in the 1970s. Early work followed the now familiar pattern in claiming that an attractive facial appearance had significantly favourable effects on teachers' expectations of the academic prowess of children and that attractive children behaved better than their unattractive peers. Unsurprisingly, these findings caused ripples in educational and psychological circles. However, later studies explored the findings in more depth and focused on factors such as actual academic performance, and found that the effects of appearance were attenuated, with effects more pronounced when academic performance is low. In their review, Bull and Rumsey (1988) highlighted the gap between the results of studies using photographs as stimuli and those carried out in real-life situations. They concluded that the relationship between facial appearance and actual academic performance and behaviour was weak at best. In addition, the effects relate far more strongly to teachers' expectations than to actual outcomes.

### The impact of the facial appearance of children on adults, and stereotyping by children on the basis of appearance

Bull and Rumsey's (1988) review indicated that beyond the educational setting, less attractive children were expected by adults to be less well behaved and less well adjusted, but once again found little evidence to show there are actual differences. Some studies during the 1970s and 1980s showed that less attractive children were disciplined and punished more harshly than their more attractive peers, but other studies showed no such effect.

As a spin off from research on the role of appearance of children on teachers' expectations, some research focused on the emergence of appearance stereotypes in the pupils themselves, and the age at which children start to be influenced by the facial appearance of others. Children expect more attractive teachers to be more effective (Chaikin et al. 1978), but there is no evidence of an actual effect. Evidence from Dion (1973) and Rumsey et al. (1986) indicated that stereotypical inferences about the temperament and disposition of other children and adults related to judgements of facial attractiveness were expressed from the age of six or seven years onwards, although children of this age do not necessarily share the judgements of adults on what actually constitutes a more attractive face. From the age of eight onwards children make hypothetical friendship choices on the basis of physical appearance (Dion 1973), though there is little evidence that actual friendships are formed on this basis.

*Facial appearance, persuasion, advertising and employment*

Researchers in the 1970s and 1980s also turned their attention to a variety of other topics, asking questions such as whether the facial appearance of a communicator has any effect on his/her persuasive power over an audience. Sigal and Aronson (1969) and others published research suggesting that an attractive appearance did enhance the power of a communicator's message. However, studies in the 1980s showed that perceived expertise, credibility and personal characteristics were powerful moderators of this effect (Bull and Rumsey 1988).

In relation to buying behaviour, the portrayal of physically attractive people in advertisements results in greater attention being paid to the advertisements, increases the amount of attention viewers focus on the product, increases their willingness to buy and makes it more likely that they will actually purchase the product (Halliwell and Dittmar 2004).

There were early suggestions in the research literature that physical attractiveness could favourably affect various aspects of employment, including evaluations of ability, actual job status and earning power, but other factors, most notably social skills and actual ability have subsequently been shown to mediate these judgements (Bull and Rumsey 1988). Recent research has emphasized the complexity of factors involved in judgements like these but has failed to influence the now widely held perception that a youthful appearance is an advantage in the job market.

## The relative impact of different aspects of appearance

In the 1960s, a group of researchers took up the baton of the early writers to further examine what constitutes attractiveness and beauty, and the extent to which individuals agree in their judgements of these constructs. Studies in the UK by Iliffee (1960) and by Udry (1965) in the USA showed strong interjudge agreement when ranking female faces for prettiness. The gender and geographical location of respondents had little effect. In the USA social class had no impact, whereas in the UK agreement was strongest among respondents judged by the author to be 'lower' class than among those from a 'higher' class. Age had little effect other than for those over 55 years who gave more positive rankings for the more 'mature' faces. More recent studies have confirmed significant and high interjudge agreement concerning judgements of the attractiveness of full-face photographs (Langlois et al.

2000). But the question remained as to what constitutes this attractiveness upon which people agree.

Bull and Rumsey's (1988) review showed that the mouth, then eyes, then hair followed by the nose correlated most strongly with ratings of full-face attractiveness. They also reported a consensus that the neonate features of large eyes, small nose, large mouth and small chin correlated with more positive judgements of females. Studies (however limited) have also examined the effects of eye colour, pupil size, glasses, beards, hair and dental appearance. Shaw (1981) and others found that variations in dentofacial appearance (prominent, crowded, missing teeth) have signficant effects on the impressions formed by others of people depicted in photographs and concluded first, that this may represent an important social disadvantage, and second, that parental desire to have dental anomalies corrected in their children is therefore well placed. Even though people rate dental appearance as likely to be very important in real-life situations, few studies have examined whether this is the case, with those that have (for example, Rutzen 1973) reporting minimal effects. Other factors clearly play a part: Shaw (1981) also varied background facial attractiveness and found this to have a strong effect on ratings. In relation to the wearing of glasses, Argyle and McHenry (1971) showed that the initial effects on the reactions of others are eliminated as additional information about the wearer becomes available during an interaction.

By the end of the 1980s, some researchers were grasping the nettle of the complex interplay between the reactions of others to a person's physical appearance, and the effects of these reactions on self perceptions. The vogue for work relating to impression formation, the reciprocal nature of social interaction and self-fulfilling prophecies lead several researchers (including Hatfield and Sprecher 1986; McArthur 1982) to propose a process through which stereotyped expectations ('attractive people have more desirable traits') lead people to behave differently towards attractive and unattractive people, resulting in the behaviour and differences we expect. Once elicited, this behaviour may be internalized into the self-concepts of the stereotyped people so that they make self-attributions for behaviours that were situationally induced. Although the process is more complex and involves additional factors, this framework has proved a useful heuristic with which to explore the links between appearance, social behaviour and self perceptions.

The early 1990s saw the publication of two landmark meta-analyses both of which went some way to acknowledging the complexity of the processes involved in interpersonal perception. Eagly et al. (1991) found evidence for correlations between physical attractiveness and various positive traits, but concluded that the average magnitude of the beauty-is-good effect was moderate . . . certainly not extremely strong, and the strength of the effect varied considerably from study to study. They also highlighted that effect sizes depended crucially on the type of inference participants were asked to make, and on the methodology employed by the researchers. Feingold's review (1992) concluded that physically attractive people were viewed by others as having more positive personality and social traits; however, there were 'generally trivial relationships' between physical attractiveness and measures of ability.

Throughout the 1990s, the industry which had grown up around appearance research continued to grow and flourish. The debates concerning the pervasiveness and power of the effects of physical attractiveness continued to rage among psychologists, sociologists and social commentators. In an attempt to offer a definitive view, Langlois and colleagues (2000) published a series of 11 meta-analyses. They concluded, first, that observers generally agree about who is and who is not attractive, and that levels of cross-cultural agreement in these judgements are high. Second, they reported that attractive children are judged by strangers to have more social appeal, to be better adjusted, and have higher levels of interpersonal competence than their unattractive counterparts. Similarly, attractive adults are judged to be better adjusted and to have better social and occupational competence than their less attractive peers. Third, Langlois and colleagues reported that attractive children and adults are treated more positively by others; and lastly, that physically attractive people actually exhibit more positive traits and behaviours than less attractive children and adults. It should be noted however, that Langlois et al. were less critical of the methodologies of the studies included in their meta-analyses than their forerunners, Bull and Rumsey (1988) and Eagly et al. (1991).

From the 1960s to the 1990s the psychology of appearance was largely the domain of social psychology. More recently, psychologists from this sub-discipline have turned their focus towards the way in which people use visibility as one of the means of performing and presenting identities (Frith and Gleeson, personal communication). This area of research proposes that people engage in self-presentation within a set of culturally defined hierarchies. These position people in a 'pecking' order according to how particular aspects of their appearance such as size, shape and skin quality fit against what is regarded as socially desirable. One's position in this hierarchy is fragile. A change in health status which has an impact on appearance can result in a sudden and dramatic shift. However, a person's status is also to some extent negotiable. People can actively engage in the process of change, or help themselves to feel better about their position in the hierarchy and a number of physical (surgery), behavioural (diet, exercise) and psychological activities can be employed to renegotiate a position. Gleeson and Frith (personal communication) have pointed out the paradoxes of this societal economy. While we may at times enjoy the pleasures of being seen and recognized, we can also be acutely aware of the scrutiny, appraisal and judgements of others. The impact of a society in which some bodies are valued more than others has been explored most thoroughly through research in the area of body image.

*Research on body image*

Research output from psychologists and sociologists interested in the concept of body image was more evident during the twentieth century than work focusing more explicitly on the impact of physical appearance. In the early 1900s, clinicians expressed the desire to understand phenomena such as phantom limb pain (Cash 2004). Initial work was sporadic; however, as the century progressed an increasing number of researchers and writers took up the baton. Schilder carried out a number of studies in the 1920s. His work culminated in the publication in 1935 of the book *The Image and Appearance of the Human Body*, in which he argued ahead of his time, that body image is not just a cognitive construct, but one also affected by the attitudes and interactions with others (Grogan 1999). Fisher and Cleveland published *Body Image and Personality* in 1968, with remarks about 'normal' and 'psychiatric' patients based on projective techniques – exploring among other things, how people assign meaning to body parts, and the basis of distortions of body perceptions. Their approach reflected the psychodynamic tendencies of the time (Pruzinsky and Cash 2002).

Although pockets of research continued over the years, it was not until the 1990s that it reached a critical mass. Until then, the bulk of research had been dominated largely by the interests of clinical psychology and psychiatry, with a particular emphasis on eating disorders in young women. However, the more general applicability of body image research was highlighted by large-scale surveys such as one by Cash et al. (1986) who reported that in a nationwide study in the USA, only 7 per cent of women expressed little concern with their appearance. Rodin et al. (1985) coined the phrase 'normative discontent' to describe the widespread dissatisfaction women have with their appearance. In addition, the growing predominance of cognitive behavioural approaches in the 1980s and the growing influence of feminist perspectives resulted in a prolific increase in the number of studies. These were drawn together in Cash and Pruzinsky's landmark volume *Body Images: Development, Deviance and Change* in 1990.

Since then, academic and clinical interest in body image has continued to grow (Grogan 1999). Although the majority of work has focused largely on the body shape and size concerns of women, reflecting the headline concerns apparent in the general population, latterly, an increase in interest in the body image concerns of men has become evident as the male body has gained visiblity in popular culture (Lee and Owens 2002). In their 2002 volume summarizing the state of play in this area, Cash and Pruzinsky picked on three main themes. First, the evidence that from early childhood onwards, body image plays an integral role in understanding many aspects of human experience; second, that it is a multi-faceted construct, defined in many different ways (Thompson et al. (1999) listed 16 definitions calling 'body image' a sponge phrase, absorbing many different connotations and meanings); and third, that there is a dearth of integration between the research emanating across and within disciplines.

Most researchers now conceptualize the body image construct as a continuum, with levels of disturbance ranging from none to extreme. Higher levels of disturbance are usually associated with other symptoms, for example, anxiety, depression and impairment in social functioning (Rumsey et al. 2004), and low levels of dissatisfaction are associated with positive adjustment and wellbeing. From the perspective of health psychology, it is interesting to note that Thompson et al. (2002) report that low to moderate levels of body image dissatisfaction and disturbance might conceivably be beneficial – leading to 'healthy' exercise and eating patterns.

Despite this increase in research in the field of body image by a group of social and clinical psychologists, the early reluctance of the majority of psychologists to engage with the pervasive nature of the psychological ramifications of appearance and body image remains. Although over the years it has become more acceptable to discuss the potential benefits of attractiveness, it remains less palatable to talk directly about the disadvantages of being unattractive or ugly. However, a third area of research has gradually gathered momentum, and a small number of health and clinical psychologists have engaged with the task of understanding the psychosocial effects of living with an appearance which is visibly different from the norm.

### The emergence of a literature on the psychology of disfigurement

In a pattern similar to the pioneers of body image and appearance research, a few early studies hinted at the need to understand better the ramifications of disfigurement. Abel (1952) noted that all of her sample of 74 patients hospitalized for corrective surgery thought their facial disfigurement was in some way a deterrent to successful living. Many complained to her of discrimination in work and social situations.

During the 1960s, there was an increasing realization among US plastic surgery teams that the majority of their patients had problems with social encounters and relationships. Sporadic publications during the 1960s and 1970s flagged up that despite the increasing sophistication in surgical techniques, all was not well in relation to the psychological adjustment of people with visible differences. Their observations were interpreted using the dominant psychodynamic perspective of the time.

The medical sociologist, Frances Cooke MacGregor (1974) noted that of all the concerns she had within the field of physical disability and rehabilitation, the greatest for her was the large number of people with disfigurements who seemed to be 'marginal' or 'forgotten' people. The increases in technical ability to alter facial appearance in the 1980s led a number of professional groups, including surgeons and dentists, to ask for evidence relating to the potential impact of these changes with questions such as: 'is it worth breaking someone's jaw to achieve a more satisfactory bite and more aesthetically pleasing profile?' Some researchers responded by trying to quantify the boundaries of an 'acceptable' and 'unacceptable' physical appearance by devising measurements of facial form. Using data derived from X-rays of faces, Lucker and Graber (1981) attempted to assess the acceptability or otherwise of protrusions of the lower jaw and lower teeth in relation to the rest of the skull, protrusions of the upper jaw and upper teeth relative to the rest of the skull, and in females, the size of the upper face and the width of the face from a front-on view. Berscheid (1986) noted that a further impetus to research was provided by the increasing culture of litigation, which led lawyers to ask questions about evidence for the impact of disfiguring injuries (for example, burns to children wearing flammable nightclothes; savage dog bites and so on). Would self-esteem be affected; would the disfigurement influence their marital and job prospects?

Small numbers of researchers in the USA and the UK responded to the increasing interest in the psychological sequelae of visible difference. Early studies were subject to sampling biases (comprising in the main, patients who were actively seeking treatment for their appearance – and in some studies, those who could afford to have elective plastic surgery. See Chapter 2). There was also an over-reliance both on case studies and small samples of people with particular conditions (for example, pockets of research concerning 'dental appearance' or 'port wine stains'). During the late 1970s, 1980s and 1990s, a critical mass of clinical psychologists working in the USA (most notably Broder, Richman and Kapp-Simon), secured employment in the field of cleft lip and palate and craniofacial anomalies. They generated influential studies exploring the adjustment of affected children, motivated in part by the desire to demonstrate the need for the inclusion of psychological services as part of a comprehensive approach to care.

In the UK, the few pockets of research that existed in the 1980s comprised studies exploring the detail of the difficulties experienced by people with disfigurements. Ray Bull's research group focused on unpicking the mechanisms of interpersonal encounters involving people with disfigurements in the hope that their findings might lead to effective ways of alleviating the problems. Their work also reflected the vogue in social psychology during the 1970s for studies of non-verbal communication and altruism. The group demonstrated that people used aspects of personal space to put a greater distance between themselves and a person with a facial difference (Bull and Stevens 1981; Rumsey et al. 1982), and also that most people avoid a social interaction with an affected person if possible. However, the altruism story was more complex. Once an interaction had been initiated, other people tended to help a person with a disfigurement more than they would the same person without a disfigurement (see Bull and Rumsey (1988) for a review). In the course of their research, Rumsey, Stevens and other co-workers took the parts of confederates appearing either with or without simulated facial disfigurements. The experience was immensely powerful, and led them to appreciate much more graphically both the impact of the reactions and behaviours of others and the role of their own behaviour on the course of social encounters.

Rumsey also noted the ideas of MacGregor, who in 1974 had proposed that in responding to others, those affected by disfigurements tended to adopt one of three strategies . . . first, a tendency to withdraw from social interaction (the 'ostrich technique'); second, a tendency to display overt hostility; and third, a tendency to be excessively charming and active, thus taking control of an encounter. Strenta and Kleck (1985) created a situation in which participants believed they were appearing to others with a facial scar applied using make up. All those who believed they were 'scarred' (in some cases the scar had been removed without the participant's knowledge) became preoccupied with their appearance, felt it was affecting their interactions and believed they could sense a strong reactivity to their disfigurement from others. To explore this further, Rumsey designed a study in which the presence or absence of a disfigurement, and the level of social skill were varied. The most positive reciprocal communication and the most favourable impressions were formed by participants responding to the person made up to be visibly different in the skilled condition, and the least to the same person when visibly different and lacking in social skill. Although this was a laboratory-based study, it represented a promising finding. Until then, the overwhelming message in disfigurement research had been a negative one, with a heavy focus on problems and difficulties. The task of tackling the insidious biases in society towards those with an attractive physical appearance and replacing the 'beauty myths' with attitudes more inclusive and accepting of diversity in physical appearance seemed a mountain too high to climb quickly. The finding that the behaviour of the affected person could be a strong influence on the outcome of social interaction led to a subsequent trail of research examining the potential of social skills training as an intervention for those affected.

In the UK, two events around 1990 galvanized subsequent research into disfigurement. The first was a chance meeting between two psychologists (Richard Lansdown and Nichola Rumsey) and a plastic surgeon (David Harris) at a surgical conference in Cambridge. The three ruefully discussed the lack of attention, research funding and care provision for those with visible disfigurements. They made plans to convene a multidisciplinary group of like-minded people, and the Disfigurement Interest Group was founded. This group was in existence for eight years and met regularly to exchange ideas, present ongoing research findings, and latterly to write and publish a book, designed to offer health care professionals an authoritative account of current knowledge about the problems and issues in the field of visible disfigurement and of ways of adapting health care to more closely meet the needs of patients (Lansdown et al. 1997).

Following the King's Cross underground station fire and subsequent publicity about the resulting burn injuries, James Partridge (1990) published a book called *Changing Faces*, charting his experience of recovery following an extensive burn injury ten years previously, when he was 18. Nichola Rumsey and James Partridge (then a cow farmer living on the small Channel Island of Guernsey) met during the launch of this book and exchanged insights and findings. Partridge discovered that researchers had begun to grapple with the trials and tribulations of living with a disfigurement and subsequently read Bull and Rumsey's book *The Social Psychology of Facial Appearance* (1988). Nichola in turn read James's book *Changing Faces* and discovered that the eloquence of a person with a disfigurement was considerably superior to an academic with a research interest in the topic! The reaction from many members of the public to Partridge's book convinced him that although the surgical treatment of burns had advanced in the decade since his accident, psychosocial care was still notable by its absence. He decided that action was needed to address this all too evident need, and established a charity to promote the cause of those affected by disfigurement. James Partridge agreed to include some core funding for research in his fundraising plans and the charity Changing Faces and the Changing Faces Research Unit were established in 1992. The small research team focused on the development and evaluation of social interaction skills interventions and other services offered by the charity, and acted as a catalyst for the activities of the Disfigurement Interest Group. The clear focus of the research on identifying needs and designing and evaluating interventions to meet these needs led to an obvious home for this research within the newly emerging discipline of health psychology. Since their inception, both the Charity and the Research Unit have undergone considerable expansion. *Changing Faces* now offers a raft of both direct and indirect methods of support and intervention, and exerts a considerable influence in the development and implementation of changes to health care provision and policy (see www.changingfaces.org.uk). The Research Unit became a free-standing centre (The Centre for Appearance Research) in 1998, and at the time of publication has a core membership of 35 researchers.

In the USA and the UK, the 1990s saw further efforts to describe and understand the problems associated with a visible difference, and to examine the similarities and differences between the experiences of those with different conditions. Researchers from the disciplines of sociology and nursing made significant contributions to the burgeoning literature. Michael Hughes, a social worker, published a book, *The Social Consequences of Facial Disfigurement* (1998), based on his studies of people with disfigurement caused by cancer or trauma. Rob Newell published *Body Image and Disfigurement Care* in 2000. Aimed at health care professionals, this text was based on Newell's research with people with head and neck cancer and a range of other disfigurements. He offered readers a thorough appraisal of the strengths and weaknesses of previous research, and examined the potential of the fear-avoidance model of coping as a framework within which to understand the difficulties of those affected. Both authors joined the swelling band of researchers who were highlighting the deficits of the prevailing biomedical model of care in meeting the psychosocial needs expressed by those affected. However, despite the gathering body of research and the increasing number of personal accounts charting the social and psychological problems, care provision has remained focused on medical and surgical interventions (see Chapter 6). The subtext is an exclusive focus on enhancing appearance, with the effect that the role in adjustment of additional social and psychological factors is minimized. For those progressing to treatment, a medical or surgical 'fix' is offered as the answer to presenting problems. This limited health care agenda also has the effect of reinforcing pre-existing societal biases that favour physical attractiveness and pathologize visible differences.

By the end of the 1990s, there was a coherent body of research highlighting the extent of individual variation in adjustment, and confirming the lack of a relationship between the extent and severity of a disfigurement and levels of distress (Lansdown et al. 1997). The effect of type of condition, and demographic variables such as gender and age also had less impact than many had previously expected, and a number of psychological factors began to emerge with increasing regularity in research findings as contenders for the most influential variables in the multifactorial process of adjustment (see Chapters 4 and 5).

Around this time, researchers also become aware that in their efforts to chart the problems and difficulties, they too had been guilty of pathologizing rather than normalizing disfigurement. In the last few years there has been a growing movement both in the USA and the UK to broaden the focus of research to those who cope well – to learn from the positives as well as the difficulties. Attention has turned to factors promoting resilience in disfigurement, reflecting developments in other areas of psychology. As Seligman and other proponents of the positive psychology movement argue, the glass half empty approach had permeated psychology and the other behavioural sciences for too long.

A second recent trend for researchers in disfigurement has been to highlight the similarities and differences in appearance-related concerns for people with and without objective disfigurements. Previously, there was an assumption that the problems experienced by many people with disfigurements were unique to them; however, the recent increase of research into the appearance and body image concerns in the general population (see Chapter 3), together with an appreciation of the extent of variation in adjustment within the population of people with disfigurements (see Chapter 5), has highlighted the many similarities in concerns across the population spectrum.

In 1997, a British plastic surgeon Gus McGrouther, commented that legislation exists to counter prejudice and discrimination on the grounds of race, disability and age, and ruefully noted that disfigurement had become the 'last bastion of discrimination in the UK'. The chance of legislation to reduce discrimination on the basis of physical appearance appears remote. The research community engaged with the task of understanding and meeting the needs of those affected by appearance concerns is alive and kicking, but appearance-related research remains a minority sport and specialist knowledge in this area is the preserve of a few. In view of the pervasive nature of appearance concerns in the population, it is time that health psychologists grasped the nettle and acknowledged the role of these issues in the adjustment and wellbeing of many.

## Chapter summary

♦ Humans are fascinated by faces. There are examples of high levels of interest and investment in facial appearance since records began;

♦ In westernized nations, current levels of investment (behavioural and financial) in physical appearance are high despite the lack of evidence that beauty and attractiveness are linked with happiness;

♦ We make stereotypic judgements of people's attributes (for example, character and occupation) on the basis of external appearance;

♦ People with visible disfigurements frequently report that their appearance evokes negative responses from others;

♦ Research into the psychology of appearance was initially the preserve of a few. The momentum grew in the 1970s and 1980s, and appearance was linked by researchers to a wide range of benefits. By the 1990s, it was clear that the early findings painted an overly simplistic picture;

♦ Body image research has focused in the main on weight and shape concerns. It is generally accepted to be a multifaceted construct playing a part in a broad range of human experiences;

♦ Research on the consequences of disfigurement during the 1990s charted both the problems and the clear lack of service provision to meet the needs of those affected;

♦ In their efforts to explain individual differences in adjustment to disfigurement, researchers have begun to focus on factors contributing to positive adjustment to visible difference;

♦ There are considerable degrees of overlap in the distress experienced by people troubled by their appearance whether or not they have an 'abnormality' of appearance.

## Discussion points

♦ Is society's obsession with appearance greater currently than in previous eras?

♦ Why do people make stereotypic judgements on the basis of appearance? Where do these stereotypes come from?

♦ Are attractive people more socially competent than their less attractive counterparts? If so, why?
♦ How would you react when encountering someone with a serious facial disfigurement such as a burn? Why would you react in this way?

## Further reading

Cash, T.F. (2004) Body image: past, present and future. *Body Image*, 1: 1–5.
Davis, K. (1995) *Reshaping the Female Body: the Dilemma of Cosmetic Surgery.* London: Routledge.
Etcoff, N. (1999) *Survival of the Prettiest: The Science of Beauty.* London: Little, Brown and Company.
MacLachlan, M. (2004) *Embodiment: Clinical, Critical and Cultural Perspectives on Health and Illness.* Maidenhead: Open University Press.

CHAPTER
2

# The challenges facing researchers in the area

*(with contributions from Alex Clarke, Hannah Frith and Kate Gleeson)*

Over recent years, the body of literature relating to psychological aspects of appearance has burgeoned. While this is clearly an increasingly popular topic of investigation, new and established researchers alike have been confronted by an array of methodological and professional challenges, some of which are specific to appearance research while others are also relevant to other areas of health psychology. Recognition of these difficulties is not new. More than a decade ago, Strauss and Broder (1991) reviewed the problems with research into the psychosocial aspects of cleft palate and related craniofacial conditions. Many of the issues they identified apply to appearance research more widely and, regrettably, it seems that many are still relevant today.

In this chapter we refer to both published literature and our own research experience, with the aim of providing a practical and constructive aid for anyone embarking on research into the psychosocial aspects of appearance. We begin by highlighting issues that warrant careful consideration for any project, regardless of methodology, for example the researcher's underlying assumptions about appearance, the sensitive nature of the topic under investigation, problems with recruitment and funding. Two challenges especially demanding in this field are the valid integration of evidence from different types of sources (for example, different methods and methodologies) and the development and testing of appropriate and useable theories and models. We therefore highlight difficulties relating to the choice of measures, critically consider the theories and models that are available to underpin research in this area and suggest a new framework to guide future activity. Finally, we propose that the range of research methods being used in this area should be broadened.

## Underlying assumptions

Before embarking on work in this area, it is important to realize that much of the existing research has been based on two suppositions. First, that the needs and concerns of those individuals with an objective, visible disfigurement are different to those without. This has led to the development of two distinct literatures (see Chapters 3 and 4) but there are many similarities between these populations and the variation within either group is as broad as it is between them. A challenge facing researchers is how best to investigate the nature and impact of appearance issues among those with or without a visible difference in a way that preserves the uniqueness of their situation without ignoring the commonality. Researchers are faced with many of the same issues, irrespective of which group they are studying. It may therefore be more useful in the future to focus on the questions being asked and the challenges facing the researcher as opposed to a segregation of the populations under investigation. Second, issues such as social anxiety are deemed by the uninitiated to be experienced by all those who have some kind of visible difference, and distress is presumed to be greater among those with a larger or more noticeable disfigurement. These assumptions have encouraged the development of a pathological, problem-focused approach to research, with more positive experiences often being overlooked.

## Sensitivities around appearance research

Appearance can be a very sensitive and emotive topic and some individuals (including those who scrutinize applications for funding or ethics approval) might envisage participation in this research as stressful. Participants who are distressed by their appearance may find it upsetting to describe or reflect upon their experiences and it is possible that standardized measures, if not chosen carefully, could exacerbate this distress. With this in mind, it is imperative to establish clear protocols for referring participants on for further support where appropriate and to ensure they are aware of relevant sources of help, for example through charitable organizations, condition-specific groups or health care services (see Chapter 6).

While much of the research in this area has focused on problems and difficulties in relation to appearance, it is interesting to note that individuals might be equally sensitive or wary of reporting positive aspects or satisfaction with their appearance. Attempts to manage our appearance and visual selves occur in a context dominated by the message that you cannot, and indeed should not, judge a book by its cover (Frith and Gleeson, personal communication). This can make it difficult for people to talk about appearance issues. A person who is visibly different may be counselled by well-meaning others that it is the person within that counts, making it difficult for them to admit to being bothered by their appearance. These supposed words of reassurance overlook the fact that appearance *is* important to them:

> I don't believe my friends see through to the real me, they just see ME, which is *all* of me. People who are close to me don't like me *despite* my appearance or even because of it – I am one package!!!! I feel the same way about myself; I like me – *all* of me.
>
> (Bates, personal communication)

Interestingly, an evaluation of a camouflage makeup service (Kent 2002) reported that a response rate of only 33 per cent was partly due to concerns about appearing vain or preoccupied with appearance and a sense of shame. Indeed, one person in Kent's study specifically asked not to be sent the follow-up questionnaire for fear that their housemate might open the post and thereby know they had been to a camouflage service.

This creates problems for the researcher interested in appearance concerns because it may be difficult for participants to honestly admit distress about physical features in the face of pressure to deny their significance and the implication that their concerns are shallow and trivial. This was evident among women with an early-stage pre-invasive breast condition (DCIS) (Harcourt and Griffiths 2003) who reported finding it difficult to discuss concerns about their appearance when they felt they should be grateful that the treatment had possibly saved their lives. It is sometimes difficult for researchers to move beyond participants' assertions that appearance is unimportant in order to explore any genuine concerns (Frith and Gleeson 2004). Yet such research evidence concerning both positive and negative aspects of appearance is needed if a truly informed, comprehensive understanding is to be achieved in order to inform clinical care.

## Research funding

The number of researchers working in this field seems to be increasing and the competition for research funding is intense. No doubt most health psychologists will argue that their specialist area suffers from insufficient research funding. Our experience suggests that securing funding for appearance research is especially difficult since stakeholders who effectively shape research agendas may not see this as a priority area. When resources are at a premium, there is a danger that appearance issues are pushed aside to make way for more 'worthy' concerns. Yet we believe it is only by raising the applied and academic profile of appearance and disfigurement and by making funders aware of the extent and effects of these issues that they will attract the necessary funding. It might appear to be a Catch-22 situation but we are hopeful that this situation is amenable to change. Indeed, we have recently been greatly heartened by a decision by the Healing Foundation (a charitable organization) to fund a significant stream of research into the psychosocial aspects of appearance with a focus on ultimately improving the lives of individuals affected.

## Sampling and recruitment

One could be forgiven for assuming that since everybody has an appearance of some kind, accessing and recruiting participants into appearance-related research would be straightforward and trouble-free. Unfortunately this is not the case and sampling and recruitment in this area is often problematic and presents two particular challenges: access and quantity.

There may be obvious sources of participants if the research focuses on a specific population, for example adolescents. Yet it is possible that any method of recruitment is more likely to attract individuals who have greater interest in issues pertaining to their appearance. It may be that 'resilient' individuals who place less importance on it are less likely to volunteer participation. One possible solution is for researchers to use a range of recruitment strategies and to continue to investigate alternative methods of promoting their work.

Some groups may seem harder to recruit than others. For example, concern has been raised (see Schwartz and Brownell 2004) over the tendency for appearance research to be dominated by female participants. Several researchers have noted difficulty in recruiting males (Wallace, personal communication) and it has been speculated (Dittmar et al. 2001) that this may reflect their reluctance about discussing appearance and body image issues. However, Frith and Gleeson (2004) suggest that they are not reticent, but choose to talk about appearance in a different way than women do. For example, when researching men's use of clothing, participants would on the one hand deny taking an interest in their appearance but then proceed to describe how they manipulated and managed their choice of clothing in response to how they felt about their body. Clearly this presents challenges to researchers who need to find ways of engaging male participants.

### Recruiting participants from a range of cultural and ethnic groups

Most appearance-related research to date has been conducted in western cultures, in particular the USA and the UK and with individuals with a good command of the English language since few standardized appearance measures have been translated. Very little research has explored the experiences of those from differing cultural and ethnic groups but this may be particularly pertinent since issues of disfigurement, stigma and shame may be culturally bound (Papadopoulos et al. 1999b). Researchers need to focus on recruiting participants from a more varied range of ethnic groups and establishing studies specifically into these issues. Research within the Centre for Appearance Research (CAR) has repeatedly had an over-whelmingly white/UK sample despite our attempts to recruit participants from clinics with catchment areas of large, mixed ethnic populations. This has led us to believe that there may be other factors at play that result in individuals from some ethnic groups not attending clinics at which appearance issues may be evident (for example general plastics or derma-tology). It could be that for some reason they are not referred or that they do not seek help in relation to appearance concerns. Clearly this is an issue for further research and requires other means of reaching these individuals, possibly through community leaders as opposed to health care systems.

*Student samples*

Too much of the existing research has relied upon student samples, par-ticularly when examining appearance and body image among individuals without a visible difference and in the development of body image measures. Alternative means of identifying and contacting participants are clearly needed. For example, Halliwell and Dittmar (2004) have demon-strated how snowball sampling using email contacts enabled them to recruit 202 non-student women across a range of demographic variables in order to study the impact of media advertising on body-focused anxiety.

*Recruiting people with a visible difference*

Recruitment is by no means easy for researchers seeking participants whose appearance is different to 'the norm'. For practical, logistical and ethical reasons, participants for condition-specific research are typically recruited through relevant support organizations at a national, regional or local level (Cochrane and Slade 1999; Papadopoulos et al. 2002); hospital or clinic contact (Beaune et al. 2004; Fortune et al. 2005; Hughes 1998; Kent and Keahone 2001; Thompson et al. 2002; Wahl et al. 2002); or a combination of both (Hill and Kennedy 2002; Moss and Carr 2004a). These can offer ready access to the targeted group, but there are problems with recruitment via hospital sources or support groups. First, it limits the research to those who are in contact with health care professionals and/or seeking some kind of intervention or support. This may give an emphasis to the acute phase of appearance-altering conditions (Thompson and Kent 2001). Second, the psychosocial variables (for example, the perceived social support) that might influence whether or not individuals have contact with such organizations might also be influential in determining levels of psychosocial adjustment. Hughes (1998) describes his difficulty in gaining access to individuals with congenital disfigurements since surgeons were concerned that introducing a research element into their care could jeopardize the doctor–patient relationship. This demonstrates possible problems if health care professionals are acting as gatekeepers for recruitment into research and if the only source of recruitment is through hospital contacts.

We currently know little about those individuals whose appearance is visibly different but who do not seek treatment or support. This group is likely to include those who could be considered 'well adjusted'. Recent emphasis upon resilience and positive outcomes (see Chapter 5) suggests this group will become a focus of future research. One of the challenges facing researchers is to identify appropriate ways of accessing these individuals, possibly through the use of advertising, the media or snowball sampling. For example Martin and Newell (2004) successfully recruited 366 participants from both hospital clinics and through the media in order to investigate the factor structure of the Hospital Anxiety and Depression Scale (HADS) for use among people with a visible difference.

Often research in this area has small sample sizes because of the variability in the incidence, aetiology, severity, location and permanence of a visible difference. For example, Papadopoulos and colleagues' (1999a) evaluation of a CBT (cognitive behavioural therapy) intervention involved a total of 16 participants (eight in both the control and intervention groups). Although this was sufficient to meet their requirements for statistical power, researchers have often blamed insignificant results and low levels of psychological problems and dysfunction upon small sample sizes and methodological failings (Eiserman 2001). This implies that problems are undoubtedly present but have not been detected because the methods and measures were unsuitable or inadequate. On the contrary, it is possible that such problems are just not being experienced to a high degree, even in a larger sample. The challenge facing researchers is how best to investigate the factors that distinguish between those who do or do not experience such distress and how best to offer appropriate support to whose who do.

Given the difficulties surrounding recruitment generally, there is a danger that rarer conditions may be overlooked since recruitment may be deemed especially problematic. For example, port wine stains are estimated to occur in 1 in 3000 births (Sheerin et al. 1995), the incidence of scleroderma is 1 in 5000 (Joachim and Acorn 2003) and Treacher Collins Syndrome affects less than 1 in 25,000 (Beaune et al. 2004), so obtaining a large sample might be both a difficult and lengthy process. However, high response rates among people with rarer conditions suggest they are often highly motivated and keen for their voices to be heard. Researchers may be pleasantly surprised by patients' willingness to participate, especially if they feel that issues around appearance are typically overlooked. For example, Vamos (1990) reported that patients with rheumatoid arthritis were pleased that interest was being shown in the appearance aspects of their condition in contrast to the usual biomedical focus on physical pain and functioning. Similarly, research conducted in clinic settings by members of CAR has typically gained very high response rates. For example, an audit of the appearance-related concerns of outpatients had a response rate of 86 per cent (Rumsey et al. 2004).

Good response rates have also been evident in studies that have required considerable involvement by participants. For example, 72 per cent of participants in a prospective study of women's experiences of breast reconstruction took part in data collection on three occasions over one year (Harcourt et al. 2003). Similarly, recruitment among burn-injured patients is often considered difficult but investing considerable time in developing and maintaining a good rapport with participants and a flexible approach towards the timing of data collection has enabled a response rate of more than 66 per cent in a detailed examination of the psychosocial needs of this group (Phillips, personal communication). We take these experiences as further evidence that appearance is a pertinent issue for many patient groups and that, despite concerns that focusing on such sensitive topics can be upsetting, they are willing and keen to participate.

*Multi-centred research*

One possible means of increasing sample sizes is to conduct multi-centred research. For example, a study of individuals attending 15 different out-patient clinics in Bristol and London identified the levels of distress among a total of 458 people with a range of appearance-altering conditions (Rumsey et al. 2004). Ongoing collaborative research by members of CAR in Bristol and research teams in the USA is enabling the investigation of quality of life among adolescents with a variety of craniofacial conditions and our work with colleagues in London, Sheffield, Bradford and Warwick is enabling the recruitment of more than 1500 participants with a variety of appearance-altering conditions. The difficulty is that significant differences might be evident in reports from participants recruited through different sites. For example, patients seeking elective plastic surgery in London-based clinics have reported exceptionally high levels of anxiety and depressive symptoms compared with patients attending a comparable clinic in Bristol (Rumsey et al. 2004). The reasons for such variations in participants' reports, experiences and levels of psychosocial wellbeing might only be surmised but could reflect differences in systems of care or health care professionals' attitudes towards appearance issues. While multi-centred studies do enable a quantitative comparison that may identify the most appropriate care provision, this would ideally require a sample size from each site sufficiently large enough to be statistically significant.

## Conceptualizing participants as a homogenous group

From the outset, a researcher must decide whether it is appropriate to focus on appearance and disfigurement issues *per se*, or whether their research is to concentrate on one specific condition (for example, cleft palate) or population group (for example, adolescents). The conceptual shift towards the study of disfigurement or appearance as a phenomenon independent of medical condition has a number of benefits. For example, it may be advantageous in terms of the application of findings and provision of care aimed at addressing issues (social anxiety for instance) deemed common to all, regardless of the cause of disfigurement (see Chapter 7).

Yet there are equally strong arguments against amalgamating a range of conditions within a study or single intervention group and for not viewing individuals as a homogenous group. Although there is remarkable consistency in the kinds of problems reported by people with different conditions (Partridge et al. 1997; see also Chapter 4 of this volume), it is important that factors that predict distress in one condition are not assumed to be predictive in others. Combining different diagnostic groups has already been raised as an issue among cleft-palate research. For example research may combine individuals with cleft lip, cleft palate, combined cleft and uni-lateral or bi-lateral cleft (Strauss and Broder 1991). Likewise, categorizations such as 'dermatological conditions' fail to identify the unique experiences of those with differing diagnoses within this group (see Porter et al. (1986) in Chapter 5 of this volume). The decision as to whether to combine groups needs to be addressed in the early planning of a research study and by reference back to the aims of the research.

These problems of sampling and recruitment are clearly illustrated by our experiences as members of a collaboration of researchers who have joined together to investigate the following question: 'What is it that distinguishes between those who adjust well to disfigurement and those who experience problems?' This involves a large-scale survey of more than 1000 participants from hospital clinics and hundreds more from primary care and community samples in order that the findings are not only applicable to individuals currently in the health care system or diagnosed as having one particular condition. The process of agreeing a sampling frame for this study was arduous. Eventually it was decided to use a $2 \times 4$ sampling frame in terms of (a) whether a disfigurement was normally visible to the public or not; and (b) the aetiology of the visible difference (congenital, trauma, disease or other). Breaking down the sampling frame further according to demographics, the site of disfigurement and specific condition would have been too cumbersome and costly to fulfill, despite having considerable resources at our disposal. While not ideal, the final sampling frame will enable the investigation of adjustment to disfigurement *per se* yet still allow useful sub-comparisons to be made. Furthermore, a series of smaller subsidiary studies will enable particular issues and populations to be followed up in depth.

In order for different patient populations to be studied together (as in the aforementioned example) then there must be a way of drawing meaningful comparisons between them (for example, the severity of acne scarring with the severity of facial palsy) and also a clear justification for this comparison. One of the problems facing researchers is the measurement of the relative severity of a disfigurement (see Chapter 5). If perceived severity is one of the most important variables in studying the psychosocial impact of any appearance-related change, it is important not only to know whether it is a term that is meaningful in a psychological sense but that it can be measured in a reliable and valid way. In many studies, judgements based on size, location and visibility all contribute to a rating standardized by inter-rater agreement. Thus, while it is widely reported that severity of a disfigurement does not predict psychological distress, this is a finding that is perhaps less convincing from studies between groups with a variety of disfigurements (Robinson et al. 1996), than from studies within groups having a unitary medical condition (Love et al. 1987; Malt and Ugland 1989). A further difficulty in combining heterogenous groups with various appearance-altering conditions is the potential impact of associated dysfunction with some conditions, particularly where disfigurement affects the face (for example, head and neck cancer). Others, for example dermatological conditions, are less likely to impinge upon function.

There is also a danger that population (as opposed to diagnostic) groups are seen as homogenous with similar experiences of, and attitudes towards appearance. For example, it is short sighted to assume that all adolescents will be troubled by their appearance or that older people will not (Johnston et al. 2004; Spicer 2002). Indeed, Spicer (2002) concludes that older people have often been excluded from appearance-related research for this reason. Similarly, assuming that individuals necessarily view ageing as having a negative impact upon appearance and that this is worse for women than for men, fails to understand their differing experiences across the lifespan (Halliwell and Dittmar 2003). Meanwhile some groups have been the focus of very little research – for example, changes to appearance brought on by the menopause have received little attention (Banister 1999).

## Comparison and control groups

Evaluations of interventions for people with appearance-related concerns have often been made without the use of a control or comparison group (Kleve et al. 2002). It is therefore, perhaps more appropriate to view these as very useful and informative audits rather than research. Choosing an appropriate comparison group presents the researcher with further dilemmas and the literature is peppered with examples of research without comparison groups or of questionable associations having been made. For example, Beale and colleagues (1980) compared breast augmentation patients with ENT (ear, nose and throat) patients on the premise that the comparison group was undergoing non-cosmetic surgery. However, ENT surgery (as indeed all surgery) does have the potential to impact upon appearance, which may be a concern for the patients involved.

**Timing of data collection**

Given that individuals may already be experiencing considerable concern over their appearance it is imperative that participation in research does not exacerbate such distress and is not overly burdensome or time consuming. Wherever possible it will be advantageous to coordinate research involving individuals in the health care system with the time schedule and overall delivery of care. For example, data collection around the time of surgery might be inappropriate given the possible heightened levels of anxiety and may require compromises being made towards the perceived methodological rigour of the research.

Timing of data collection can be especially relevant in some situations, such as among people treated for life-threatening conditions (for instance cancer) or severe burns. Phillips (personal communication) found that parents of burn-injured children were reluctant to take part in research while their child was in hospital since they did not want to leave their child for any period of time. However, they were very keen to participate in in-depth interviews once their child had returned home and the imminent threat of the burn had subsided. Indeed, appearance-related concerns are likely to become more pertinent over time as threat to life subsides, contact with hospital staff and other patients reduces and patients start to compare themselves and their appearance with healthy peers (see Gamba et al. 1992; Pendley et al. 1997). Furthermore, they may only feel it is appropriate to discuss and acknowledge appearance concerns once the immediate threat to life has diminished. However, it is important not to assume adjustment to an altered appearance invariably improves over time – it is more appropriate to view it as a continual stressor which will at times be exacerbated or allayed by experiences.

As in other areas of research, timing can be especially pertinent for researchers aiming to evaluate a new intervention or service (be it surgical, psychological or educational). New services and procedures take time to establish and initial teething problems may need to be rectified. Therefore, an early-stage evaluation might not truly reflect the intervention as it matures, yet failure to include a psychosocial evaluation from the outset could result in the widespread take up of surgical or supportive interventions that do not offer the anticipated psychosocial benefits. Furthermore, availability of new procedures and changes to provision of care during the timespan of a study may mean that what was once considered the most favourable treatment may have been superseded by the time the research is completed and published. For example, Reaby (1998) and Reaby and Hort (1995) examined women's experiences of breast reconstruction up to seven years after surgery, during which time developments in surgical processes and care would have taken place.

Data collection might also be influenced by the time of year. For example anxiety could be heightened when warmer weather makes it harder or uncomfortable for individuals who are troubled by their appearance to disguise it under make up or clothing and when some activities deemed as threatening such as going to the beach, swimming and so on are more likely to take place. Furthermore, some dermatological conditions may be exacerbated by certain weather conditions (Papadopoulos et al. 1999b), while other causes of disfigurement increase in incidence at particular times of the year. For example, burn injuries resulting from barbecues and camping fires tend to increase over spring and summer months. In recent years there have been attempts to reduce the incidence of burns injuries associated with firework celebrations around Guy Fawkes' night (5 November) in the UK. However, in 2003, 1136 firework injuries were still reported around this date, 588 of which involved children and adolescents under 18 years of age (Department of Trade and Industry: www.dti.gov.uk).

## Context of data collection

The visibility of some disfigurements such as dermatological conditions may be influenced by the immediate context in which data collection takes place (e.g. air conditioning, room temperatures or anxiety about a clinic attendance), which may influence data relating to perceived visibility of a condition. Similarly, an individual's self-reports might be influenced by their recent social context and the extent to which they are upwardly or downwardly comparing themselves with others (see Chapter 5), and the experience of being in a clinic setting with others with a similar condition might encourage such comparisons to be made. It is therefore imperative that the situation/context is understood in any assessment of evaluative or affective states (Cash 2002b) and that state (as opposed or in addition to trait) measures are used in assessment when appropriate (Thompson 2004).

## Research methods

Increasingly a wide range of methods are being used within appearance research, ranging from lab-based studies to applied clinical settings and using both qualitative and quantitative approaches.

### Experimental, lab-based research

Lab-based studies might sometimes be criticized for lacking ecological validity and paying little attention to sociocultural influences, yet experimental research has provided valuable empirical evidence and a better understanding of the problems reported by people with a visible difference. For example, work on proxemics, or interpersonal distance, has demonstrated that the subjective experience of social interactions can be objectively studied (Rumsey et al. 1982). In a series of studies in both controlled natural and laboratory settings, levels of face-to-face contact and social interaction have been varied in ways that would be impossible in a 'real life' setting. Rumsey and Bull conducted a series of studies using make up to manipulate the presence of a facial disfigurement on an individual without a visible difference to provide experimental evidence to support personal reports that people with a visible disfigurement are often avoided by others (see Chapter 4 for more detail). Such evidence could not be obtained if a within-subjects design had not been employed, enabling direct comparisons on the basis of the presence or absence of a disfigurement without the confounding influence of factors such as gender, social skills or other aspects of appearance.

Studies using make up have also demonstrated that merely expecting a negative response is enough for a visibly different person to perceive and report social interactions differently. For example, participants who were led to believe that they had a false facial scar attributed negative reactions and interactions with others to prejudice towards their unusual appearance (Kleck and Strenta 1980; Strenta and Kleck 1985; and Chapter 1 of this book). In fact, the cosmetic scar had been surreptitiously removed and the participants in Kleck and Strenta's research did not look visibly different. Clearly such manipulation is only possible with a controlled, experimental design and a degree of deception. These findings have provided a clear rationale for psychological treatment strategies and led to subsequent research providing evidence that since social skills are a better predictor of successful functioning than disfigurement, social skills training is a logical intervention (see Chapter 7).

Controlled, experimental studies have also enabled the systematic investigation of the impact of the media on body-focused anxiety and body image satisfaction. Research in this area has a strong applied focus given recent concerns by sources such as the British Medical Association (2000) over the use of very thin models in the media, increases in reported body dissatisfaction and the incidence of eating disorders. Halliwell and Dittmar (2004) used computer imaging software to manipulate the size of models used in deodorant advertisements. While the 'attractiveness' of the models remained constant, their images were stretched in order to appear as either 'thin' (UK size 8) or 'average' (UK size 14). Results demonstrated that exposure to a thin model was associated with increased body-focused anxiety among women who internalized sociocultural ideals of thinness and appearance. The study suggests that body-focused anxiety could be reduced by the use of average-sized models and that such advertisements would still successfully promote the product. These findings have clear implications for the advertising industry and suggest that interventions focusing on lowering levels of internalization of sociocultural attitudes towards appearance could be beneficial. Possible ways of doing this and the effectiveness of such interventions have yet to be examined (see Chapter 7). Future research might try to embrace technological developments that could enable images in television advertisements to be manipulated in a similar manner and could also investigate the impact of 'average' as opposed to 'perfect' facial appearances. However, experimental research into the impact of the media has been criticized (Grogan 1999) for low ecological validity since it is conducted in unfamiliar settings where participants focus specifically upon an advert, so the results may not represent the impact of the media in participants' normal environment.

### Measuring attractiveness

The notion of 'attractiveness' has proven very problematic to researchers. Much early experimental research used photographs of 'attractive' and 'unattractive' people, but clearly attraction consists of more than physical features. Systematic measurement of the human face and body (see Roberts-Harry (1997) for an overview of anthropometric measurement techniques) does not equate to an assessment of attractiveness, yet still attempts are made to computer-generate representations of supposed 'perfect' faces. Interestingly, such images are typically rated as 'boring'. Clearly a subjective concept such as attraction requires subjective assessment.

### Self-report studies

Much existing research into the psychosocial impact of disfigurement is reported within the medical literature and consists largely of surveys and descriptive studies investigating specific medical conditions such as burns (Wallace and Lees 1988), port wine stains (Lanigan and Cotterill 1989) and vitiligo (Porter et al. 1986). Often the focus is on the psychosocial aspects of the condition and appearance issues are seen as a subsidiary issue. For example, research into the psychosocial impact of cancer among adolescents has given surprisingly scant attention to issues of appearance, yet many adolescents report the changes to their appearance being the most distressing aspect of the disease and its treatment (Eiser 1998; Rowland 1990).

Some of the clearest descriptions of the problems faced by people who are visibly different are found in self-report data. Personal accounts such as that of Partridge (1990) have been very influential in stimulating the academic study of altered appearance and raising the profile of the problems they encounter, yet case studies have received relatively little attention as a research method.

The majority of the research in this area has been retrospective, quantitative, cross-sectional and correlational. This is problematic because while participants may describe their current feelings and concerns about their body and appearance, they may not be able to portray their actual past experience and may misrepresent both positive and negative experiences. It is also likely that cognitive dissonance may be in operation, leading individuals to adjust their earlier view of themselves in order to reconcile their previous and present situations. This is evident in research among women who have undergone reconstructive surgery after a mastectomy (see O'Gorman and McCrum 1988; Reaby and Hort 1995). In addition, recent events and the research setting may influence an individual's perceptions and self-reports (see above). In essence, 'the body is a moving target' (Cash 2002b: 41) and thoughts about appearance change over time and throughout a lifetime. State reports of appearance or body image are not necessarily constant from day to day or during a single day. However, despite fluctuations, people may restore homeostasis between current (state) and trait body satisfaction. A study by Melynk et al. (2004) required 108 American college students to respond to the Body Image States Scale (BISS) (Cash et al. 2002) twice daily for six days and found a correlation between trait satisfaction with appearance and reports of state body image.

*Longitudinal research*

There is a pressing need for longitudinal research to explore the dynamic, fluctuating nature of adjustment and to examine the issues relevant to significant points across the lifespan. For example, cross-sectional research (Sheerin et al. 1995) found that children with port wine stains were not particularly bothered by their appearance yet adolescents and adults were. Prospective, longitudinal research could identify when and how such issues become pertinent, especially among progressive conditions such as vitiligo. This would have clear implications for the delivery of age-appropriate care and also enable possible links between stress and skin conditions to be established.

Within the non-disfigurement literature, longitudinal research has tended to focus on body dissatisfaction and weight (Heatherton et al. 1997; Rizvi et al. 1999), with recent studies focusing on adolescent populations (Holsen et al. 2001). Wholly prospective, longitudinal research among individuals with a visible disfigurement is often very difficult. Pre-intervention surgical or medical data collection is feasible (for example, to evaluate the psycho-social impact of treatment among people with port wine stains (Hansen et al. 2003) or psoriasis (Fortune et al. 2005)) but it is often impossible to collect pre-disfigurement, baseline data. Prospective research (Dropkin 2001) has examined the relationship between anxiety and self-care among 75 head and neck cancer patients due to undergo surgical treatment. The fifth post-operative day was usefully identified as being a significant point in their acceptance of their altered appearance. However, patients were only followed up for six days post-operatively and longitudinal follow up is needed. Even if pre-surgical baseline data is collected, as in this example, it is likely that the process of undergoing and receiving a diagnosis will have already impacted upon patients' thoughts and feelings about their body. This has been evident in current research examining women's experiences of chemotherapy. In interviews conducted prior to the start of treatment, women have described how their expectations of its impact upon their appearance are already influencing their appraisal of their current appearance (Harcourt and Frith, personal communication).

In an ideal world, much research would benefit from employing a longitudinal and prospective design with recruitment and data collection taking place throughout the year. However, discrete data collection points within a longitudinal study, for example at six-monthly intervals, might still overlook periods that were especially significant for individuals concerned and longitudinal research does place particular demands on both the researcher and the researched. Repeated involvement in a longitudinal study could itself influence individuals' thoughts about appearance. Rusch et al. (2000) conducted a longitudinal study involving parents of 57 children who had sustained traumatic injury that necessitated plastic surgery. Almost all (98 per cent) were identified as suffering post-traumatic stress disorder (PTSD), anxiety or depression within five days of the injury occurring. One month later this had reduced to 82 per cent and to 44 per cent at 12 months. Rusch and colleagues suggested that the frequent research interviews were seen by many parents as an informal intervention which could have increased their vigilance or likelihood of talking to their child about psychosocial issues. This raises the question as to whether the situation captured in a research setting is ever equivalent to that beyond it.

Finally, longitudinal research is also needed to consider the longer-term effectiveness of psychosocial interventions. While Robinson et al. (1996) evaluated a social interaction skills training programme and included a six-month follow up there is a paucity of research that has considered any longer-term implications of care.

### Randomized controlled trials (RCTs)

The case for the use of RCTs in today's climate of accountability and evidence-based practice is strong and convincing (see Robson (2002) for a review). Health clinicians, managers and policy makers are used to evaluating the effectiveness of treatments and interventions on the basis of RCTs, thus research conducted in this way may be more acceptable to this audience and prestigious medical journals. While health psychologists (especially those working in an applied health context) must be aware of the value of RCTs they should also be mindful of the debates concerning their applicability in psychosocial care (Bottomley 1997; Robson 2002). We believe that much careful thought is needed before an RCT is used to evaluate the impact of care relating to appearance.

Specifically, even though it is comparatively easy to control and standardize drug treatments within an RCT, appearance-related surgical and psychosocial interventions present a host of different problems. Individual differences such as variations in scarring (e.g. the tendency to develop keloid scars) cannot be controlled but might influence the objective and subjective outcome of appearance-related surgery which may or may not be an influencing factor upon adjustment (see later chapters).

Most importantly, RCTs take away patient choice about their treatment and presume individuals to be merely passive responders as opposed to conscious, interactive participants (Robson 2002). In essence, they are only given the choice about whether or not to enter the trial – they have no input in active decision making about their treatment. This can be especially pertinent when an RCT is used to compare the psychosocial impact of surgical procedures with differing cosmetic outcome. For example, Dean et al. (1983) employed an RCT to compare the psychological impact of delayed versus immediate breast reconstruction among women undergoing a mastectomy for breast cancer. In this instance, randomization meant that women were leaving decisions about their future physical appearance effectively to chance. This increased the likelihood of a biased sample since those women wanting to take a more active involvement in decisions about their appearance or with a preference for or against reconstruction would be unlikely to risk being assigned to the alternative group. Hence the findings of the research might only be applicable to a sub-set of patients who have no particular preference about their treatment. However, the suitability of an RCT in this particular study must be considered in relation to developments over time in respect of what is considered acceptable ethical practice. More recently, an RCT was deemed appropriate in order to compare the psychosocial impact of three different methods of delayed breast reconstruction (Brandberg et al. 1999). In this instance, all participants had made the initial decision to undergo some kind of delayed reconstruction involving the transfer of their own tissue from a donor site elsewhere on their body. Brandberg and colleagues state that participants were keen to be randomized, supporting the suggestion that patients may not want to be faced with making the decision about the intricacies of procedures (Deber et al. 1996).

Finally, an RCT used to evaluate a psychosocial intervention tells us very little about why that intervention is beneficial or otherwise. Reported improvements could be a result of the content of the intervention, the way it is delivered or, in the case of group interventions, the opportunity for contact with other individuals with similar concerns. In essence, it tells us nothing about context and process. Also it may be impossible for researchers and others (that is to say those facilitating a psychosocial intervention) to be blind as to which condition an individual was allocated (Papadopoulos et al. 1999b). More sophisticated designs and assessments are needed to unravel and identify which aspects of an intervention are proving helpful.

However, despite having raised many reservations we would not want to dismiss the use of RCTs. It has proven useful, for example in evaluating a leaflet offering cognitive-behavioural guidance to people with facial disfigurement (Newell and Clarke 2000). There is a danger that, without evidence from well-conducted, prospective RCTs, then current surgical techniques may be superseded by newer procedures without any evidence of their psychosocial benefits. An RCT may prove invaluable as one of a number, as opposed to the sole, component within a programme of research (Robson 2002). An ongoing challenge for researchers is to ensure that the RCT is used where appropriate with caution and that robust alternatives are developed.

## The multiplicity of variables implicated in adjustment

In many instances, research alludes to adjustment to appearance but as yet it is unclear precisely what factors are implicated in this process. The list of variables that may play a part in determining individual differences is extensive and includes social support, coping, self-esteem, attributional style and investment placed on appearance (Moss 1997; see also Chapter 5). However, research including all these variables would be burdensome on the participant and necessitate a large sample in order to claim statistical power. Difficult choices have to be made as to which variables to include and which to omit.

Similarly, quantitative research requires an appropriate outcome measure and again the literature indicates a wide range of possibilities, in particular anxiety, body image and quality of life. While numerous measures of each of these constructs exist, two of the most widely used are the Derriford Appearance Scale (DAS) and the Hospital Anxiety and Depression Scale (HADS) (see Box 2.1).

These outcomes are often used to indicate adjustment, but exactly what do we mean by the term adjustment in this context? Often it is not clearly defined in research studies. Is it an outcome or a process? Are we referring to low levels of distress or high quality of life? Or could it be defined as not seeking further treatment to 'improve' appearance? If we take this last view, how do we explain the situation reported anecdotally by health care professionals, in which people who might previously have been deemed well adjusted seize the opportunity for new and possibly pioneering appearance-enhancing surgical procedures?

Since the psychosocial impact of appearance is so complex, it seems inappropriate to measure one or two elements in isolation. A balance is needed between comprehensive assessment and an excessive battery of questionnaires, yet researchers are faced with several dilemmas. First, the constructs under investigation, for example body image, are typically complex and many researchers have failed to explicitly state which definition or

> **Box 2.1   Examples of questionnaires often used as outcome measures in appearance research**
>
> ◆ The Derriford Appearance Scale (DAS-59) (Carr et al. 2000) and the short-form DAS-24 (Carr et al. 2005) centre on the notion of 'self-consciousness of appearance' and have increased the potential for reliable measurement of adjustment to appearance. Ongoing research should provide an extensive database of normative data for clinical and non-clinical groups for this scale. This will be beneficial since normative data for many outcome measures are often lacking or is based on unrepresentative, white student populations (Strauss and Broder 1991).
>
> ◆ The Hospital Anxiety and Depression Scale (HADS) (Zigmond and Snaith 1983) is relatively brief (14 items), easy to complete and, importantly, has proven popular among health care professionals who appreciate the use of 'cut-off' scores to identity individuals who might benefit from further psychological support. The psychometric properties of the HADS have been contested but a recent favourable review (Bjelland et al. 2002) has supported its use. Martin and Newell (2004) concluded that the HADS is an effective tool for use among people with a visible difference but called for further research to investigate whether it is more appropriately viewed as being a tridimensional measure of depression, anxiety and negative affectivity rather than merely anxiety and depression.

aspect of the construct is their focus (see Thompson (2004) and Thompson and Van den Berg (2002) for an overview of problems with body image assessment).

Second, generic measures of psychosocial functioning may fail to tap into the specific issues pertinent to appearance (for example social anxiety as opposed to anxiety in general). Recognized measures can also be criticized for relying on the researcher's assumptions about appearance and thereby fail to gain the participant's perspective (see below for consideration of the use of qualitative methods). Many measures lack acceptable levels of reliability and validity (White 2002) although advances are being made in this area. For example, the Body Image Scale (Hopwood et al. 2001) has undergone psychometric validation and appears to be a useful, reliable measure of body image in women with breast cancer. Thompson (2004) has offered a helpful list of advice for researchers and clinicians selecting a tool to measure body image.

Despite these limitations, clinicians and researchers are still engaged in the quest for the elusive 'holy grail' of a quantifiable way of assessing the psychosocial impact of appearance (see Ching et al. (2002) for a review

of 34 instruments including widely used measures such as GHQ and
Rosenberg's Self-Esteem Scale). Ching and colleagues point out that 'psychological' measures have low face validity with respect to measuring
aesthetic surgery outcomes. However, these scales assess a wide variety of
psychological constructs and are not necessarily intended to be appearance-
specific. Ching and his co-workers rate the Derriford Appearance Scale
(DAS) highly in terms of good content, face and predictive validity but in
line with other measures, its assumption of morbidity and pathology goes
against the call for equal emphasis on the positive aspects of appearance (see
Chapter 5). Also, such measures could be ambiguous in that a person's
prevailing concerns about appearance might or might not relate to the
obvious condition or 'disfigurement' for which they are receiving treatment.

Likewise, how can we be sure that outcomes such as anxiety or depression
are necessarily due to appearance concerns related to the condition under
investigation? People with a visible difference are not immune to problems
with relationships, work, finances and so on and it would be inappropriate
to attribute reported levels of distress to the visible difference. Standardized
measures typically assess major variables but the disfigurement might only
be a specific, narrowly defined aspect of a person's life (Koo 1995). Some
quality of life measures specifically include an appearance dimension. For
example, the European Organization for Research and Treatment of Cancer
(EORTC) has devised a quality of life instrument that includes a body
image subscale for breast cancer patients and the WHOQOL (World Health
Organization Quality of Life Questionnaire) also includes appearance. The
development and use of such measures is one way in which the appearance-
related impact of medical or surgical developments are considered but there
is still a way to go before appearance issues are given the prominence that is
currently given to quality of life generally.

One approach to overcome the problems of suitable measures has been
the development of a flexible methodology (see Rumsey et al. 2004). This
has involved use of recognized, standardized measures supplemented by
visual analogue scales (VAS) developed and tested in order to quickly and
easily assess issues such as satisfaction with social support that are deemed
important and for which there are no suitable measures.

## Theories and models

A major dilemma is the choice of appropriate models and theories to guide
and underpin research in this area. This has proven problematic because
the available models are typically limited in scope or incorporate dimensions that cannot be easily measured. Until recently we have avoided using
any particular theory or model because, given the multiple factors contributing to adjustment to appearance, it felt too soon to be constraining our
thinking about the factors that should be included. However, exploratory

research has now provided such a plethora of knowledge about the mass of variables implicated in individuals' experiences and adjustment (see Chapter 5) that it now feels necessary to marshal this list of variables into a manageable format. We feel that theories and models are useful in a constrained and specific context but remain uneasy with the choice and frameworks currently available. We are also aware that it is all too easy to allocate a 'tag' of process or outcome to some concepts within these models (for example, coping) whereas in different contexts these can be either or both.

We now briefly overview some of the key theories and models available to researchers in this area. We have classified these into three categories: those used within health psychology more widely; generic appearance or body image theories and those that are condition- or treatment-specific. We have chosen examples rather than attempt a comprehensive overview. When contemplating the choice and use of these or any other frameworks it is important to bear in mind what situations and processes they are trying to represent and whether this is pertinent to the specific research question. For us, a useful model should:

♦ acknowledge individual differences in appraisals and reactions to appearance;
♦ be applicable to individuals with or without a visible difference in order to normalize appearance issues;
♦ allow for positives as well as negatives;
♦ be amenable to a range of research methodologies;
♦ have a practical application as opposed to being solely academic.

### Models used within health psychology more generally

Health psychologists have employed a variety of models to examine why individuals do or do not engage in a wide range of health behaviours, many of which have a direct impact upon appearance. However, appearance is rarely the focus or motivation for such research and indeed it may be over-looked entirely. Individuals do not engage in health behaviours solely for health-related reasons – wanting to 'look good' or change appearance can be a strong motivator. A recent survey of 687 people aged 11–21 years confirmed that appearance is an important motivation for or against healthy living in terms of diet and exercise, especially among females (Haste 2004). In particular, concerns about appearance were frequently cited as reasons for not exercising: more than one quarter did not exercise because they were unhappy with the way they looked in exercise clothing. According to Leary et al.:

> certain people need to and want to exercise but do not do so because of concerns with the impressions they make while exercising. People who perceive themselves to be overweight, scrawny or disproportioned may

be reluctant to be seen bouncing around in an aerobics class, swimming
at the local pool, jogging in public or lifting weights.

(1994: 466)

Many health behaviours result from people's attempts to manage the
impression they create to other people (see Leary et al. 1994). For example,
despite being aware of the possible risks of skin infections, HIV transmission
and hepatitis, adolescents felt it was acceptable for actors and singers to sport
a tattoo (Houghton et al. 1995). Although, interestingly, they felt that tattoos
on a teacher would be inappropriate. It seems individuals may be prepared
to risk the chance of developing serious health problems (coronary heart
disease or cancers) because they worry about gaining weight if they were
to give up smoking. Indeed, having cited examples including steroid
use, cosmetic surgery, tattooing and dieting, Leary et al. claim that 'self
presentational motives are often so strong that they lead people to engage
in impression-creating behaviours that are, in the long term, dangerous to
themselves or to others' (1994: 461).

Models used in appearance research and health psychology research
more generally include social cognition models, self-regulatory theory and
theories of stress and coping. We now consider these in turn:

*Social cognition models*

The use of social cognition models is illustrated by health-promotion
campaigns concerning the dangers of sun exposure, in which the health
messages contradict attitudes towards the attractiveness of suntans. Castle et al.
(1999) used the stages of change and health belief models (HBM) in an
intervention aimed at young women's suntanning behaviour (see Chapter 7).
Similarly, the HBM was also used by Carmel and colleagues (1994) to
investigate the role of age in predicting protective behaviour while in the
sun. They found that the value placed on appearance (and health) were the
best predictors of likelihood to engage in sun exposure protective behaviour.

A limited number of studies have used social cognition models to
examine aspects of treatment and health care intervention that have clear
appearance implications. For example, Searle et al. (2000) used protection
motivation theory as a framework for a qualitative study investigating
children's adherence to eye patching as treatment for amblyopia (decreased
vision where no physical cause is apparent). The appearance and noticeability of the eye patch were cited as reasons against patching among
older, but not younger, children. Clearly this is useful information for health
care professionals working with this population and demonstrates the
importance of appearance in relation to treatment adherence.

Yet while these social cognition models may help to explain some
appearance-related behaviours, they are often inadequate when trying to
understand the complexity of individuals' experiences of living with

appearance-related concerns or disfigurement. First, perceived subjective norms included in some models (for example, the Theory of Planned Behaviour) clearly have an influence upon whether or not an individual will attempt to change their looks or engage in health behaviours that may impact upon appearance. However, these models view individuals as acting rationally and under their own free will but people who feel pressured to conform to societal and media standards of appearance may feel unable to act under their own volition. Meanwhile individuals with a visible disfigurement may claim they act in response to other people's reactions to their appearance as opposed to their own free choice. These models give insufficient attention to the social and cultural context in which an individual's experiences are located and fail to consider the complexity of social interactions that are imperative in appearance. They also fail to incorporate the key variables that are likely to influence adjustment (for example, the importance of appearance to self-concept). Furthermore, given the dynamic nature of 'adjustment' any comprehensive theory or model should incorporate a process of appraisal and feedback if it is to have a useful role in understanding appearance concerns. Individuals will not always feel the same about their appearance and those who are deemed to be 'well adjusted' may not always remain so (Thompson et al. 2002). Relevant and useful models must allow for this fluctuation and change.

*Self-regulatory theory*

Leventhal's dynamic, self-regulatory model (Leventhal et al. 1980) has informed the investigation of a variety of appearance-related conditions, for example, psoriasis (Fortune et al. 2000) and vitiligo (Papadopoulos et al. 2002). It seems reasonable that individuals' beliefs concerning the consequences, duration, cause, seriousness, curability and identity (label and symptoms) of a visible difference might influence distress and behaviour. However, it has been suggested (Cochrane and Slade 1999) that some constructs such as time line or curability are inappropriate for conditions such as cleft lip among adult populations when no further treatment is available. Also, while this framework might be appealing as a guide to research among people with a visible difference, how relevant is it among people who do not have a visible difference? Furthermore, the framework encompasses the notion of coping which itself is fraught with problems relating to conceptualization and assessment.

*Theories of stress and coping*

Various theories of stress and coping have been employed widely in this area. In particular, Lazarus and Folkman's Transactional Model has been used, focusing on individual appraisals of stressors and coping strategies in relation to appearance (see Cochrane and Slade 1999; Dropkin 1989).

Dropkin (1989) used this approach to explain post-operative recovery and adjustment to an altered appearance among patients treated for head and neck cancer. 'Successful' adaptation required individuals to change their personal value system and to place less reliance upon appearance. The advantages of this model are that appraisal and coping are seen as influencing one another (hence the model can be considered dynamic); it considers both positive and negative aspects and offers a potentially useful framework for clinical intervention.

Most studies based on Lazarus and Folkman's model have focused on identifying strategies deemed adaptive (e.g. seeking social support) or mal-adaptive (e.g. avoidance) in relation to adjustment to appearance. For example, Hill and Kennedy (2002) investigated the role of coping strategies in mediating subjective disability in people with psoriasis. This cross-sectional study found that most of the variance in distress was predicted by venting of emotions, alcohol and drug use ideation and mental disengage-ment (all deemed maladaptive). However, strategies found to be maladaptive in one situation might be useful elsewhere and what is effective for one individual might not be so for another. For example camouflage make up might be useful in the short term or for a specific situation but could be maladaptive if the person's social interaction is reliant upon it (see Chapter 6).

A further problem is that much of the research using Lazarus and Folkman's model has relied on the use of coping checklists, the problems with which have been discussed in detail elsewhere (see Coyne and Gottlieb 1996). In summary, such checklists are unable to represent the full range of coping strategies and behaviours and have limited use if the individual interpretation and nature of the stressor is not understood. There is a danger that research requiring participants to complete a coping checklist may view disfigurement as a single stressor, yet it is likely to involve a complex array of perceived stressors, for example dealing with the reactions of other people, concerns around treatment or adjusting to the loss of previous looks. In this vein, Somerfield (1997) suggests that research should focus on 'target stressors' – those that are likely to affect a sizeable percentage of the target population, are stressful for them and are amenable to intervention. Such research would involve a series of studies examining a range of specific appearance-related stressors pertinent to those affected. For example, one study focusing on coping with social interactions, while another focuses on stress of treatment. Such a programme of research would then build a detailed understanding of dealing with appearance issues. This approach has been used to explain Changing Faces' approach towards support and interventions for individuals troubled by a disfigurement (Clarke 1999).

### Appearance-related models

Early cognition models of body image disturbance focused on the discrep-ancy between an individual's perceived actual and ideal self that is activated by everyday events and images such as those portrayed in the media. For example, Thompson et al. (1999) review a number of models of body image and describe the process by which an individual's thinking becomes more and more dominated by negative thoughts and appraisals of their appearance. Ultimately, any social situation is interpreted as being related to appearance (for example, the break up of a relationship or failure in a job interview) and specifically appearance-related situations are viewed negatively. Models of body image disturbance were developed in relation to eating disorders and weight dissatisfaction and while they incorporate constructs that may also be useful for research into visible difference and appearance more generally, they still need to be developed and tested in relation to a broader population.

Cash's cognitive-behavioural model (2002b) recognizes that past, historical issues (cultural socialization, interpersonal experiences, physical characteristics and personality attributes) influence the development of body image attitudes and schemas. Appearance-schematic processing, activating events, internal dialogues (thoughts and so on), body image emotions and adjustive self-regulation strategies and behaviours (such as avoidance, appearance self-management) are seen as being influential in the present. All aspects are deemed to influence one another – there are no arrows to indicate any direction of causal relationships or influences because of the complexity of the issue and interactions between the variables. The advantage of Cash's model is that it is dynamic in recognizing that current, proximal influences will become historical influences in the future and although developed in the context of body image research it could apply both to individuals with or without a visible difference. It can also explain both positive and negative body image as opposed to the predominantly negative focus of much research and theorizing. The framework incorporates some highly complex processes (self-schema, self-regulatory processes and coping) and contentious constructs (personality), making testing of the whole model difficult and onerous but it remains a very useful aid to guide research and needs further empirical testing.

Although many theories of body image have been developed, until recently there has been a paucity of models and theoretical frameworks specifically relating to disfigurement. Perspectives on stigma (Goffman 1963), shame (Gilbert and Thompson 2002) and social exclusion (Leary 1990) have all informed the development of a number of appearance and disfigurement-specific models, primarily with a focus on cognitive-behavioural principles (see also Chapter 4).

For example, Kent (2002) proposed a model centred around appearance anxiety and perceived stigma. Anxiety is deemed to increase when an individual is confronted by a 'triggering event' (something they perceive will draw attention to their appearance, such as going to a social or sporting event). Attempts to reduce their anxiety are deemed to focus on the use of two coping strategies: avoidance and concealment. While these might be effective in the short term, they do not address the reasons why this event was initially perceived as stressful and ultimately they serve to reinforce appearance anxiety. This model explicitly acknowledges the role of social norms and it is dynamic since the strategies reinforce anxiety, which in turn reinforces the perceived need for the strategy (in this case concealment). However, this is a limited view of coping strategies and it may be the threat (anticipation) of a triggering event rather than the event itself that raises anxiety (Heason 2003). Furthermore, this model is problem focused and the concepts that are central to the model (shame and stigma) are problematic in their emphasis on pathology (see Chapter 4).

Newell (2000a) has suggested a testable fear/avoidance model of social anxiety among people with a visible difference. He usefully proposes a continuum of confrontational and avoidant responses, as opposed to discreet categories of good or bad adjustment, with confrontation presumed to be more adaptive. Avoidance is deemed to be prompted by fear and antici-pation of a negative outcome. This leads the individual to engage in an increasingly restricted range of activities, with ever more innocuous situations determined as threatening. For example an individual may choose to exercise at home in order to avoid the perceived threatening environ-ment of a gym, or shop over the Internet to avoid clothes shops. Fear and avoidance are therefore conceptualized as possible mediators of adjustment/distress. This model offers a feasible explanation for social avoidance grounded in a cognitive–behavioural approach that has informed inter-vention strategies and clinical trials. However, it is again unclear to what extent this model accounts for the development of distress in non-disfigured populations or how or why distress occurs initially.

Recently Moss and Carr (2004) have explored the use of the multi-faceted self-concept as a means of explaining adjustment to disfigurement. Poorer adjustment is hypothesized among disfigured individuals for whom appearance is a more central or important aspect of self-concept, whose self-aspects are dominated by appearance-related information at the expense of non-appearance-related information (compartmentalization) and whose self-concept is cognitively more complex. Those who have difficulty in adjusting to their appearance therefore tend to have a negative view of themselves that is reinforced by their interpretation of information and events. The authors acknowledge that the influence of other variables such as social support and coping strategies has still to be examined and it has yet to be applied among people without a visible difference. However, this framework does identify areas for intervention that may complement existing CBT or social skills training.

In summary, there are some similarities between these models: specifically the focuses on cognitive–behavioural concepts, on avoidance and con-cealment as coping strategies and on the relative importance given to appearance. However, they have still to be tested thoroughly among populations of individuals with and without a visible difference.

*Condition- and treatment-specific models*

Some models attempt to explain appearance issues within specific condition or treatment groups. For example, White (2000) again drew upon cognitive behavioural principles to develop a model of the impact of changes to appearance among people treated for cancer. This proposes that psychological distress, negative thoughts and maladaptive coping strategies are more evident in patients who place greater importance on their appearance and whose cancer is affecting a particularly valued part of the body. However, White (2002) points out that this is not always the case and, as ever, individual differences have an important role to play. He also usefully emphasizes that investment in appearance is not constant and is influenced by time, the status of the disease and social context. While this model was developed specifically to describe issues among people with cancer, it may be applicable to other conditions and offers a useful framework for intervention. However, the model does not seek to explain what determines the importance placed on a body part.

Sarwer et al. (1997) offer a model that focuses on motivation for cosmetic surgery, in which the reality of the physical appearance, developmental (e.g. teasing about appearance), socio-cultural (e.g. ideals portrayed in the media) and perceptual (e.g. evaluation of size) factors influence body image and self-esteem. Body image valence (the extent to which appearance is important to self-esteem) is linked with body image satisfaction (value). Individuals with negative or low valence are unlikely to seek cosmetic surgery regardless of whether or not they are satisfied with their appearance. Those with high valence (who place importance on body image) are likely to seek cosmetic surgery if they feel dissatisfied with their appearance. This has yet to be investigated in detail among people undergoing non-surgical cosmetic treatment such as botox (see Chapter 6) but Sarwer and Crerand (2004) claim it is equally applicable in such instances. It seems likely that attitudes towards the surgery will also be relevant and it also remains to be seen whether this framework could also be applied to other situations, for example, altering appearance through other methods such as tattooing or suntanning.

*Using models*

It is becoming clear that while the current array of models and theories have facilitated research, they fall short of providing a comprehensive understanding of individual experiences of appearance. It has been suggested (Bond and McDowell 2001) that there is a distance between the theories used by professionals and the individual's perspective. While a range of appearance-specific models have been proposed, their success and utility are limited, as they all require further testing and refinement. Yet models do facilitate comparisons between research findings, they can guide the development of research and interventions and provide a focus for much-needed discussion and debate. New researchers to the field may find them especially helpful. However, we must not allow the models to constrain our thinking and blind us to new ideas or the complexities of the relationships among the various factors involved. A consideration of the psychological issues around selection and preparation of patients for face transplantation (Clarke and Butler 2004) illustrates the potential benefits of using theoretical frameworks when faced with a new situation in which there is a lack of previous research evidence and literature. In this instance, Clarke and Butler demonstrate how previous decision-making research derived from the theory of planned behaviour provides a guide for empirical research, although they were clearly not constrained in their thinking by the use of their chosen framework.

### A framework to guide appearance research and practice

Given the complexity of the topic, it would seem useful to identify issues that could be included as a framework as opposed to being too prescriptive. Integrating information about the development, maintenance and management of appearance-related distress within one testable framework would be very helpful for researchers and clinicians alike. To this end, the collaboration of researchers referred to previously have agreed upon a framework to facilitate investigation of appearance issues that will guide both research and the development of clinical interventions (see Figure 2.1). This framework focuses on inputs or predisposing factors, intervening cognitive processes and outcomes. While the predisposing factors (demographic and sociocultural factors) play a role in adjustment, they are difficult or impossible to change. In contrast, cognitive processes (self-perceptions, social comparisons) are more amenable to change through intervention. The framework suggests that appearance-related beliefs, influenced by predisposing factors such as cultural, aesthetic and peer group pressures, result in the

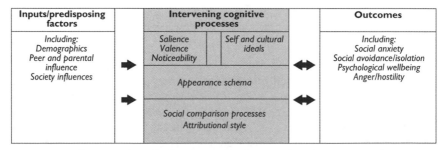

*Figure 2.1* A framework to facilitate investigations and inverventions relating to appearance concerns

commodity of physical appearance as part of the self-concept. The importance of appearance within the self-concept varies from situation to situation and over time, depending in part upon past memories and the attention given to and appraisal of the current social environment. The individual rates or values their appearance as positive or negative and again, this value is changeable. The process of self-appraisal, achieved by comparison with cultural ideals, evaluation of social encounters and subjective perceptions of the noticeability of appearance, produces beliefs about individual appearance. At the same time, processes such as attributional style, coping processes and social support influence the beliefs and value about appearance and may exacerbate or ameliorate distress. Most people will meet or exceed a subjective norm, that is to say the individual is satisfied with their appearance, or can modify it using clothing, make up and so on to enhance it to an acceptable level. Where this subjective norm is not met, people who cope positively are those who have developed strategies (such as good social skills) and re-evaluated their beliefs about the relative importance of appearance. People who place a high importance on appearance, appraise it as failing in comparison to subjective norms and employ negative coping strategies, are likely to experience poor adjustment, possibly evidenced through social anxiety, social avoidance (as described by Newell) and in some specific situations shame and hostility (Kent and Thompson 2002). Poor adjustment may also lead to a request for treatment or support. Although these aspects of the model are depicted as 'outcomes' they also influence the cognitive processing and therefore the framework is dynamic and should be construed as non-linear. A benefit of the framework is that it has potential to explain positive experiences and reports about appearance because it is not solely problem-focused.

This framework has similarities with some of the models outlined previously, for example Cash's model of body dissatisfaction. However, while Cash aims to explain body development and experiences through an amalgam of complex processes that are presented as a whole, the development of the framework outlined above has been driven by the need for a relatively straightforward guide to inform the provision of support and intervention. It therefore gives a central focus to intervention and factors that are amenable to change. Given the similarities in the nature of appearance concerns reported by individuals with or without a visible difference and the variables shown to mediate or moderate appearance-distress (see Chapters 3 and 4), this framework is potentially applicable to both groups but has yet to be tested.

In summary, a range of theories and models have been employed to try to understand individual experiences of appearance. So far, no single model stands out as offering a comprehensive framework to guide research and clinical intervention. A major challenge facing researchers in this area is the development, testing and implementation of useful frameworks that do not preclude thinking 'out of the box', such as that suggested above. One avenue to be usefully pursued in this quest is the use of a broader range of research methods than has previously been the case.

## Broadening the range of research methods

### Qualitative approaches

It has been widely suggested (Thompson and Kent 2001) that research into visible difference has relied too heavily on quantitative research that confounds cause and effect. This criticism equally applies to appearance research in the wider population. It could be argued that quantitative research reduces something as complex as the emotional and psychological reactions and experiences of living with a visible difference to a series of numbers and, in doing so, loses the personal meaning of the situation. Indeed, it has been suggested (Vance et al. 2001) that quantitative methods have not facilitated the discussion or reporting of sensitive appearance-related issues. Like many other areas of health psychology, appearance and disfigurement research suits a diverse range of methods and methodologies – the researcher's priority should be to use those that are the best fit with the situation and the questions under investigation. Support for the use of qualitative research in this area has therefore gained momentum, yet the full potential of qualitative approaches has still to be fully exploited.

We mentioned earlier how personal narratives have already played a substantial role in raising awareness of the personal impact of disfigurement (Lansdown et al. 1997; Partridge 1990; Piff 1998). These personal, qualitative accounts have shown how individuals often find positive experiences from living with a visible difference and it is from this literature that the notion of resilience within disfigurement has taken hold (see Mouradian 2001). As we stress throughout this book, identifying factors that distinguish between those who deal well or less favourably with a visible difference is an area in need of much further research and it is becoming clear that qualitative approaches can have a valuable role to play in this regard. Among the methods recently employed in this area have been interpretative phenomenological analysis (IPA) (Thompson et al. 2002), thematic analysis (Halliwell and Dittmar 2003), grounded theory (Johnston et al. 2004; Wahl et al. 2002), ethnographic analysis (Banister 1999) or a combination of approaches (Johnson et al. (2004) combined IPA with discourse analysis).

Frith and Gleeson (personal communication) suggest that one of the key advantages of a qualitative approach is that it uses techniques that provide an experience akin to everyday talk about appearance concerns that play a crucial role in the management and negotiation of the visible self and appearance. An interview may provide a better approximation to the ways in which people naturally deal with appearance than would a set of scales or measures designed to help them represent their concerns (Frith and Gleeson in press). The limitations of many quantitative measures used in this area were outlined earlier in this chapter.

Frith and Gleeson also suggest that, from the participant's perspective, discussions about appearance in an interview setting might be a more satisfying way to discuss issues that are potentially sensitive and painful and might create a more supportive and possibly empowering experience. An interview could also help people to develop their thinking, to clarify ideas that they may have never fully thought through or articulated and may also help them to bring forward detail and complexity that they would not otherwise be encouraged to share. They also suggest that qualitative methods could be useful because the well-tried and tested toolbox of traditional empirical measures requires the researcher to know the territory of enquiry very well before beginning to collect data. However, since it is not always evident what the issues will be, qualitative researchers claim that open questions gain insights that could not be achieved through other means.

Frith and Gleeson also stress that while empirical health psychology can focus on complexity at the point of analysis (once the data is collected, and often by using fairly complex multivariate techniques), qualitative research can bring a concern with process into the data collection itself. People can be asked to describe quite complex situations, explore specific contexts and make comparisons across contexts in a way which allows the researcher to examine the complexity of the range of different concerns, values and motivations that people juggle in managing appearance and presentation strategies.

Yet an increased use of qualitative approaches is not without difficulties. First, as with all appearance research, there may be dangers in encouraging participants to dwell on their experiences. This could prove distressing for people troubled by their appearance and appropriate referral routes or sources of support need to be established and easily accessible (see 'Sensitivities around appearance research' earlier in this chapter). Second, while qualitative methods may give a detailed understanding of a topic that has been previously unresearched, they do not enable generalizations of research findings. Researchers using qualitative methods may find that health care professionals and policy makers might only be confident with generalizable quantitative research and their findings may therefore have less impact on policy and provision of care. Third, they rely on the participant being able to identify and voice their experiences. In order to gain an understanding of the impact of disfigurement and other appearance issues, the relevance of a wider social group (for example, the family) is needed but the researcher may then be faced with inaccessible feelings and a multitude of communication issues that may have built up if this has been ignored or not openly discussed by the family. Indeed interview-based research among people with skin conditions has been criticized by Papadopoulos et al. (1999b) on the basis that it will only identify distress that the individual is both aware of and willing to report, while any non-conscious impact is not considered.

*Focus groups*

Whilst qualitative approaches are now used more widely, most of this research has involved interviews. There is great potential to develop the use of a wider repertoire of qualitative research methods and tools, such as focus-group research or q-sort methodology. Focus groups have been used to examine body image, weight loss attitudes and behaviours among secondary school pupils (Bond and McDowell 2001), body image among boys and men (Grogan 1999), children's and adolescents' awareness of risks associated with tattooing (Houghton et al. 1995) and the experience of living with visible differences such as scleroderma, a rare, chronic illness that can involve thickened skin and swelling in addition to considerable pain (Joachim and Acorn 2003). A potential benefit of this approach is that focus groups may provide an opportunity for interaction between individuals with similar issues. Since the success of group interventions might be due, in part, to contact with other individuals, then focus groups could be beneficial for both the participants and researcher. However, since social situations may heighten anxiety among people with appearance concerns, the invitation to take part in a focus group could itself be stressful. For some, for example head and neck cancer patients, disfigurement might also be associated with dysfunction and communication problems making it difficult to take part in interview-based research, especially if a group situation might increase self-consciousness about doing so. Chapter 7 considers the difficulty in providing group support for individuals who experience social interaction anxiety as a result of their appearance.

*Visual methods*

Visual methods also have potential for much greater use within appearance research. Previous research has often used photographs as stimulus to investigate third parties' perceptions of others' appearance. For example, on the basis of photographic images, people with facial scarring have been rated as less attractive and honest than those without (Bull 1979); experienced nurses have rated photographs of head and neck cancer patients as less disfigured than their inexperienced colleagues (Lockhart 1999) and blind assessment of 'before and after' photographs has demonstrated a positive impact of a CBT intervention on the size of vitiligo lesions (Papadopoulos et al. 1999a). Stanford and McCabe (2002) used a photography/computer technique to compare actual and ideal 'body image' and found that more than 90 per cent of participants in their study had a discrepancy between the two. Yet appearance and body image are complex, three-dimensional constructs and static, two-dimensional photographs or computer images cannot simulate a sense of body integrity, neither do they allow for the mediating effect of personality and social relationships upon people's perceptions of others (Bradbury 1993).

Photography has recently gained credence as a research tool within health psychology (see Radley 2001) but has not been used to its full potential within an appearance context. This is surprising given the visual nature of the topic under investigation and there would seem to be many potential uses and benefits. Asking participants to create a photographic record of their experiences can prompt recall of experiences in interviews and places participants in control of the process and timing of data collection. A small-scale study by Hanna and Jacobs (1993) used photography to examine how four children with cancer described health. While this did not focus on appearance, a healthy physical appearance was one of the aspects identified and the cameras were popular with the children. Clearly this could be a means of engaging children and adolescents in the research process (a problem highlighted earlier in this chapter). Similarly, research with adolescent girls (Frost 2003) has demonstrated how photography or drawings can facilitate young people's ability to discuss appearance-related issues more easily.

### Observational methods

Broder (2001) has suggested that there is a need for greater use of observational methods within appearance research in applied, clinical settings. Recordings and analysis of surgical consultations would enable a useful examination of the context and way in which appearance and body image issues are discussed, treatment options presented and decisions about treatment made. However, the process of recording could be intrusive and influence the health professional's handling of the situation and/or the extent of the patient's involvement and with increasing trends towards litigation, surgeons might be extremely reluctant for their consultations to be recorded.

### Mixed methods

Recently, the benefits of combining quantitative and qualitative approaches has received much attention within health psychology, on the grounds that the two paradigms are basically compatible and offer a pragmatic approach to social and behavioural research (Tashakkori and Teddlie 1998; Yardley 2001). In recognizing the benefits of diversity, this approach places a greater emphasis upon the research question than upon the method (Bowling 1997) while still demanding rigorous evaluation of the quality of the research (Yardley 2001). Findings from qualitative and quantitative research may not necessarily concur and it is possible that a mixed approach may produce different results from either qualitative or quantitative methods (Yardley 2001). However, together these may enable a more comprehensive understanding of a topic than is obtained through the use of only one method.

Our experience has been that the flexibility afforded by mixed methods enables us to utilize approaches to data collection and analysis best suited to the intended audience. For example, if the intention is to influence the provision of burns care it may be appropriate to combine quantitative methodologies used in medical research with qualitative approaches with which health professionals or policy makers may be less well acquainted. This qualitative evidence can be a powerful illustration and clarification of quantitative findings.

### Action research

Researchers in this area could also benefit from using methodologies that enable the individuals themselves to contribute to the development of research and theory. For example Bond and McDowell (2001) report a study of adolescents' attitudes and behaviours associated with body image that employed such a participatory methodology. In this instance, adolescent members of a focus group discussion decided upon the content of a questionnaire used with a larger audience. Similarly, Lovegrove and Rumsey (2005) describe a piece of action research in which adolescents were involved in the design and implementation of an intervention aimed at combating appearance-related concerns and bullying within schools (detailed in Chapter 7). Moves towards increased participation in health care decisions make this approach eminently sensible. Indeed the implementation of NHS Research Governance in the UK dictates that patient representatives or similar should be consulted over possible research before Research Ethics Committee approval is granted. In many instances researchers might seek the opinion of members of organizations such as self-help and support groups in this respect, but a concern is that these services might be overloaded with such requests, which may have a detrimental impact upon the time and resources available to help people seeking their support.

## Dissemination of research findings

Finally, having made appropriate and often difficult decisions in response to the many dilemmas presented in this chapter and successfully completed their work, researchers must be imaginative in the dissemination of their findings to ensure that it reaches their intended audience of health care professionals, academics and policy makers. Researchers working in applied areas such as this cannot rely solely on publication in academic journals as means of influencing practice and care. Seminars, workshops, websites and newsletters aimed at relevant staff and provided at their convenience are just some of the ways in which the impact of research findings can be maximized.

## Conclusion

We hope that this chapter has demonstrated how the many, varied and complex dilemmas currently facing researchers make this an exciting and challenging area in which to work. Although many researchers are aware of these difficulties and acknowledge any weaknesses of the methods they employ, progress has been slow. From the development of measures and models to practical and logistical issues, researchers are confronted by a succession of challenges. However, studying appearance also offers opportunities to engage in stimulating, thought-provoking and ultimately rewarding research.

## Chapter summary

♦ The psychological study of issues relating to appearance and disfigurement presents researchers with an array of methodological, theoretical and logistical challenges;

♦ This can be a particularly emotive and distressing topic and researchers working in this area need to be sensitive to such concerns;

♦ Accessing and recruiting participants can be problematic. A particular challenge for those conducting research into issues around visible difference is the identification and recruitment of individuals who are not in contact with health care systems or support organizations. Recruitment of male participants, people from a variety of ethnic backgrounds and those diagnosed as having rare visible differences can prove especially challenging.

♦ It can be useful to conceptualize appearance as a phenomenon *per se* rather than focusing on particular conditions or populations, but this approach also has limitations;

♦ Much of the research in this field has been retrospective, cross-sectional and quantitative. There is a need for prospective, longitudinal research;

♦ The context and timing of data collection needs to be considered carefully;

♦ A wide range of research methods and methodologies have been employed in this area, yet there is still scope for greater use of a broader range of research methods;

♦ While a range of models and theoretical frameworks has been used, they are often inappropriate and inadequate to capture the complexity of appearance issues. An integrative, predictive and testable framework is needed to provide a cohesive conceptual basis for the evaluation of evidence from a variety of sources and to offer clear guidance for clinical application;

♦ Despite the difficulties and dilemmas that may be encountered, research into the psychology of appearance is a stimulating, thought-provoking and rewarding topic.

## Discussion points

♦ Design a research study aiming to gain an understanding of the psycho-social impact of having a visible difference. What problems might you encounter in trying to recruit participants into your study and how might you go about overcoming these difficulties?
♦ Discuss the advantages and disadvantages of using qualitative methods in health psychology research into appearance.
♦ Why has appearance often been overlooked by health psychology research?
♦ Discuss the notion that the social cognition models that are so widely used in other areas of health psychology are inadequate to explain individuals' experiences of appearance.

## Further reading

Thompson, J.K. (2004) The (mis)measurement of body image: ten strategies to improve assessment for applied and research purposes. *Body Image*, 1: 7–14.
Thompson, J.K., Heinberg, L.J., Altabe, M. and Tantleff-Dunn, S. (1999) *Exacting Beauty: Theory, Assessment and Treatment of Body Image Disturbance*. Washington, DC: American Psychological Association.

# Appearance and image issues for those without visible differences

## Concerns about appearance

Appearance-related concerns are reaching epidemic proportions in western society, with people increasingly preoccupied, and in many cases dissatisfied, with the way they look. Body dissatisfaction has a high prevalence in the population from the age of 8 years upwards (Grogan 1999), with significant consequences for the behaviour and wellbeing of many of those affected, including engaging in dietary regimes, exercising to change body shape, social anxiety and social avoidance, the outlay of significant sums on beauty products and engaging with the risks of cosmetic surgery. Rodin and colleagues (1985) coined the term 'normative discontent' to describe current levels of dissatisfaction with appearance.

What aspects of appearance are of most concern? In the 1997 Psychology Today Body Image Survey, 56 per cent of the female American respondents said they were dissatisfied with their appearance in general. The main problems were reported to be the size of abdomens (71 per cent), overall body weight (60 per cent) and lack of muscle tone (58 per cent). Almost 43 per cent of men were dissatisfied with their overall appearance. Compared with earlier surveys conducted in 1972 and 1985, overall appearance dissatisfaction had increased from 23 to 56 per cent for women, and from 15 to 43 per cent for men.

Many aspects of the face are the focus of dissatisfaction and increasing numbers of people from a range of different backgrounds are contemplating and undergoing invasive cosmetic procedures to the face. Common interventions include blepharoplasty (eyelid lift), face lifts, ear surgery, rhinoplasty (nasal surgery), chin augmentations or reductions, and injections of collagen or botox to reduce the noticeability of wrinkles (Sarwer and Crerand 2004). Unhappiness with breast size has also been widely reported. In 1996, *Self* magazine conducted a survey of over 4000 women, and found that over half would change their breasts if they could (Grant 1996).

Although Feingold and Mazzella's (1998) meta-analysis of 222 studies concluded that females consistently report more body dissatisfaction than males from adolescence throughout adulthood, the prevalence of body dissatisfaction in males continues to rise, with recent estimates ranging from 50 to 75 per cent. A recent newspaper article based on National Statistics Health Surveys (Prynn 2004) claimed that one in four men in the UK are actively dieting 'driven by health concerns and growing anxiety about their looks'. This statistic was compared with the 16 per cent of men who claimed to be dieting in 1980. Thirty-two per cent of the men surveyed in 2004 said they were restraining their eating because they wanted to increase their self-esteem. In a survey commissioned by *Men's Health* magazine in the USA completed by 1000 readers, 75 per cent were unhappy with their body shape. Most of the respondents wanted more muscle definition. Half reported specific concerns about visible signs of ageing, including hair loss and weight gain (Chaudhary 1996). Although the readership of *Men's Health* is likely to be biased in the direction of those who invest more heavily in their appearance, these findings are supported by studies with more representative samples. Cash (1992) found that 60 per cent of men with hair loss described negative social or emotional effects resulting from balding. Liossi (2003) reported that many of the appearance concerns of men seem to relate to the prevalent media images of the desirability of the mesomorphic 'V' shape body and the associated desire to increase muscle bulk, or to be generally thinner. Demarest and Allen (2000) also noted that many men believe that women prefer a degree of muscularity in their ideal man which is far greater than they possess.

Although the majority of the early research work was carried out in the USA, it is now clear that high levels of body dissatisfaction are not only the preserve of Americans. Harris and Carr (2001) reported levels of appearance concern in a questionnaire survey involving more than 2100 adults from the south west of England stratified for age and socioeconomic background. Sixty-one per cent of women and 35 per cent of men had an aspect of appearance that concerned them. Respondents were most frequently concerned with their nose, their weight, and with a variety of skin disorders including active acne, acne scarring, psoriasis, eczema and freckles. For women, breasts and abdomens were also a common source of dissatisfaction, whereas for men, hair loss came top of the list. For 25 per cent of concerned women, and 19 per cent of concerned men, there were indications of significant levels of psychological distress and behavioural dysfunction, with disruptive effects on everyday living, work and relationships. Common difficulties included social situations in which respondents felt the particular aspect of their appearance was aversive to others. Participants reported social avoidance and feelings of isolation, beliefs that they were physically unattractive and unlovable and associated difficulties in intimate relationships. For those most affected, levels of psychological distress and dysfunction were at least as severe as levels reported by patients with objective disfigurements who were on waiting lists for plastic surgery interventions.

In Liossi's (2003) study of levels of appearance concerns among 300 young adults in Wales and the south west of England, she found that 79 per cent of young men and 82 per cent of young women indicated dissatisfaction with one or more aspects of the way they look. Liossi's participants were dissatisfied with a number of physical attributes, and although the headline concerns involved weight and shape for women, and muscularity for men, dissatisfaction with other aspects of appearance was also reported. In her sample of 177 women, 48 per cent were unhappy with the shape of buttocks and hips, 40 per cent with the shape of their thighs, and 34 per cent with a general excess of weight. Sixteen per cent disliked their noses, 13 per cent their skin, and 6 per cent reported disliking 'everything' about their appearance. For the 123 males, the greatest dissatisfaction related to a lack of muscularity in body build (42 per cent), with a large gap between this and other concerns. Thirteen per cent were concerned about their lack of height, with 12 per cent concerned about the size of their genitals. Eleven per cent were distressed with their receding hairline, 9 per cent disliked their ears, 7 per cent were unhappy with their skin, and 4 per cent disliked the shape of their noses. Liossi has joined the ranks of researchers concluding that appearance dissatisfaction is normative among the adult population.

Some commentators have responded to these recent findings by suggesting that body dissatisfaction is a relatively innocuous fact of life; however, Thompson and his colleagues (1999) have been at pains to point out that 'normative discontent' should not be considered synonymous with benign discontent. In the spirit of this sentiment, Thompson and his co-authors chose the words *Exacting Beauty* for the title of their book to reflect the negative effects that can result from the extreme attractiveness standards that currently prevail – standards which they describe as 'trying' and 'unremittingly severe'. They note that although beauty ideals have existed for hundreds of years in many diverse societies, the toll of trying to meet increasingly unrealistic standards of beauty has never been more exacting.

Appearance-related distress can manifest itself emotionally, behaviourally and cognitively. Research has focused on two broad areas: the effects on self perceptions, in particular body image and self concept, and the impact of the appearance of the person in question on the perceptions and behaviour of others, with some intrepid researchers attempting to make sense of the complexities involved in the interaction between these two broad areas.

The preponderance of research on appearance and self-perceptions has come from the 'body image' stable with the majority of studies addressing the headline area of dissatisfaction, namely, weight and shape in females. Over the years, body image has been defined in numerous ways, though it is now widely accepted to be a multidimensional construct, with physiological, psychological and sociological components. Cash and Pruzinsky (1990) suggested that the term 'body image' should be recast as 'body images' to capture the diversity of the elements. A brief history of this research is offered in Chapter 1, and recent excellent reviews of the body image literature are available in Cash and Pruzinsky (2002) and Thompson et al. (2002). Research addressing the effect of appearance on the perceptions and behaviour of others has been summarized in a review by Bull and Rumsey (1988), and meta-analyses by Eagly et al. (1991) and Langlois et al. (2000) (for more detail see Chapter 1). An overview of research findings is offered in the next section, organized by developmental stage.

## Appearance and lifespan issues

Lifespan processes are clearly influential in the development and perpetuation of appearance-related self-perceptions and behaviour patterns. The majority of research to date has explored the appearance concerns of young adults. As there are large gaps in the current research literature, this consideration of the most relevant developmental factors in relation to self-perceptions and interpersonal processes relies heavily on the body image literature.

### The early years

#### Self-processes

The beginnings of the internalization of societal ideals are apparent at an early age. In order to illustrate the pervasiveness of beauty ideals and the tender age at which these influences become apparent, Thompson et al. (1999) cite the example of a 2-year-old girl who was asked: 'When your hair grows, do you want it like your mother's hair?' She replied: 'Want hair like Barbie'. For children, dolls provide a tangible image of the body. Baby dolls are usually manufactured with large eyes and mouth, long eyelashes and small noses, and unblemished skin. The most famous and widely owned dolls are Barbie and Ken, who are manufactured to possess particularly unlikely physiques. Norton et al. (1996) scaled the dolls to adult proportions, and using adult reference groups, determined a probability of less than 1 in 100,000 of women achieving Barbie's proportions, with only 2 in 100 men built like Ken! Although research exploring the impact of playing with dolls with unrealistic physical appearances has not yet been reported, there are several known examples of grown women seeking cosmetic surgery to get closer to the Barbie image.

Gilbert and Thompson (2002) believe that the roots of body dissatisfaction are likely to be in early shaming experiences occurring around the age of 2 or 3. They believe that from this time onwards, parental criticisms and putdowns, and rejection by peers contribute to the development of a fear of negative evaluations by others and the beginnings of the belief that others see the child as unattractive.

### Responses from others

Babies with characteristically 'cute' faces (a large forehead and large eyes) receive more attention from their parents (Langlois 1986). Infants rated as attractive by adults are expected to be more likeable and are expected to be easier to care for than their less attractive counterparts (Stephan and Langlois 1984). Although definitive evidence is lacking, the possibility of differential treatment of attractive and unattractive babies in the period shortly after birth remains.

## Childhood

### Self-processes

In a review article, Smolak (2004) has noted the recent increase in research relating to younger children in response to indicators of the prevalence of poor body image in pre-adolescent children. She also points out that current knowledge is hampered by the weakness of the majority of this research in relation to the definition and measurement of constructs, by inadequate sampling and a lack of longitudinal follow-up studies (see Chapter 2).

The estimates of the prevalence of appearance-related distress in children make scary reading. Smolak and colleagues reported in 1998 that it was common for as many as 40 per cent of 9- and 10-year-old girls to be dissatisfied with their bodies. It is a methodological challenge to clarify the precise childhood stage during which body dissatisfaction becomes a problem; however, there is evidence that children as young as 5 have absorbed the cultural bias against people who are overweight, and Smolak feels it is likely that there is an awareness of these standards by age 3. Harter (1999) reported that she has established a relationship between perceptions of physical appearance and global self-esteem in children aged 4 to 7. She also noted that self-ratings of physical attractiveness systematically decline across the school years.

The large majority of children are teased and bullied, often on the basis of their appearance. The peak age at which children find this teasing upsetting is 7 or 8 years, as at this stage they have not developed the cognitive skills necessary to deal effectively with verbal attacks from others. Boys are more likely to engage in teasing than are girls. Adolescent boys also report more negative comments concerning their bodies from peers than do girls (Vincent and McCabe 2000), although girls engage in more 'fat talk' with each other than boys. Harter (1999) has noted that self-related emotions such as pride, shame and embarrassment manifest in middle to late childhood and that these emotions frequently relate to physical appearance. She also maintains that the seeds for these emotions are sown much earlier in the developmental cycle.

Other gender differences in body dissatisfaction emerge between the ages of 8 and 10 (Cusumano and Thompson 2001), with about 40–70 per cent adolescent girls reporting displeasure with some aspect of their appearance (Levine and Smolak 2002). Research on boys is lacking; however, the indications are that although most want more muscles by the age of 11, levels of satisfaction with appearance generally increase during adolescence. In contrast, levels of satisfaction among girls decrease through this period (Smolak 2004).

*Responses from others*

Research summarized in Chapter 1 indicated that children rated as more attractive by others are the subject of more positive expectations from adults than their less attractive counterparts. For example, in the conclusion of their meta-analyses of attractiveness research, Langlois et al. (2000) maintained that attractive children were judged to have more social appeal, more academic competence, to be better adjusted and to have greater interpersonal competence (see Chapter 1). The majority of the research has related to expectations formed on the basis of photographs of children. The extent and pervasiveness of similar effects in more realistic settings remains to be clarified; however, on the basis of the few studies that exist, Langlois and colleagues maintained that attractive children were the recipients of fewer negative and more positive interactions, received more attention than their peers and were the subject of higher expectations of competence. Smith (1999) reported that 75 per cent of a sample of pre-adolescent girls and boys reported regular peer-related incidents concerning their appearance (for example, unsolicited comments, staring, taunting). Attractive girls were more likely to be helped, patted and praised by their peers and less attractive girls were more likely to be hit, pushed or kicked; however, no corresponding patterns of behaviour were reported for boys.

*Parental influence*

The influence of parents on the relationship between appearance and self-esteem in childhood is thought by several researchers to be considerable. Parents generally report that they like the way their children look in younger childhood, but levels of dissatisfaction appear to grow as the children age. The majority of research evidence in this area relates to parental influence on the development of eating disorders. Studies which address aspects of appearance other than weight are currently lacking. However, Liossi's (2003) qualitative interviews with young adults have provided preliminary indications that the processes are likely to be similar. Illustrative extracts from these interviews are provided in this section and suggest that parents may either knowingly or unwittingly influence their children from infancy either through modelling their own appearance-related anxieties and behaviours, or through their attitudes towards the appearance of their offspring. Very ordinary verbal exchanges (for example, discussing the appearance of other people) can communicate the importance placed on looks, and serve to create or exacerbate the body image anxieties of family members. We have all witnessed examples of different family environments – parents who consider physical appearance all important, and insist that their children are smartly turned out for the public gaze – compared with families who take a much more *laissez-faire* approach to outward appearances:

> My parents were preoccupied with appearance and weight. They were constantly dieting, exercising and expressing dislike towards their own bodies.

In Liossi's (2003) interviews, those with high levels of appearance distress talked of a growing sense of hurt and distress about their 'defective' appearance during childhood and adolescence, and of feeling overwhelmed by the social implications of appearance in general:

> My mother gave the message that the only way I will be happy and find a man is if I look thin.

The accounts of the influence of parents from participants with high levels of appearance satisfaction were strikingly different:

> My parents taught me it's what's on the inside of a person that counts, not what's on the outside. I was raised to accept people for who they are and not what they look like, and I know that my parents were proud of who I was.

> My parents made it clear that people come in all shapes and sizes, and we need to accept everyone for who they are . . . Some of my friends at school were afraid of becoming fat. They didn't just learn this from the media, they also learned this from their parents. Their mothers were constantly dieting and expressing a desire to be thin.

Harter (1999) has also noted that in middle childhood (8–11 years), children come to internalize the standards and values of those who are important to them, and at this stage come to develop an appreciation of the values of the larger society around them. Harter also commented that although some parents communicate their disdain for societal and media values and the excessive preoccupation with make up, clothing, diets and dating, many more buy in to the prevailing norms. It is children from families that buy in to societal standards who are most at risk for appearance-related distress and dysfunction. In the words of another participant with high levels of appearance concern from Liossi's study:

> Children at a very young age are already striving to attain society's unattainable 'ideal' body image. It doesn't help that their favourite toy is probably Barbie . . . They look at her and feel that all women should look like her.

*Societal influences*

The influence of the media in these processes is thought by many researchers to be considerable. Liossi (2003) noted that by the time they have reached secondary school, many children have watched 15,000 hours of television compared to the 11,000 hours they have been in school. They have seen 350,000 advertisements, half of which stress the importance of being thin and beautiful. Magazines targeted at pre-teens and adolescent girls contain a preponderance of articles on how to 'improve' appearance, for example through dieting, exercise and makeovers. There is anecdotal evidence to suggest that girls spend more time reading magazines (Smolak 2004) and watch more 'soaps' on the television than boys. These 'soaps' tend to promote more rigid and narrow ideals of attractiveness and body build for girls than other types of programmes. Tiggeman and Pennington (1990) concluded that from an early age, children 'consume' adult beliefs relating to body image especially from visual media such as television, and are susceptible to its influence in determining beliefs concerning desirable and undesirable aspects of appearance. Smolak (2004) believes that girls are more extensively and directly affected by media images than boys, though why and how these processes occur is not yet known.

*Consequences of appearance concerns*

Smolak (2004) summarized research highlighting the impact of a negative body image on self-perceptions, the increasing prevalence of associated changes in behaviour such as dieting and exercise regimes and the existence of fantasies about plastic surgery among ever-younger children. She also noted that the assumption of most researchers is that these processes put children and adolescents at risk for the development of body image and eating disturbances in adulthood.

**Adolescence**

The significance of adolescence as a life stage has gradually increased since the nineteenth century. Notwithstanding contemporary debates about whether or not it rates as one of the most challenging life stages, the dramatic changes in body shape resulting from pubertal growth spurts can make it a potential hot-bed for appearance concerns.

The desire to blend in and to qualify as 'normal' can be a central facet of wellbeing during adolescence (Liossi 2003), and physical appearance is frequently the prime focus for evaluating whether an individual blends in with a peer group. External appearances are often perceived as the initial gateway for friendships and dating, further exacerbating the importance attached to self-presentation by those in this life stage. There is evidence that appearance concerns affect the daily life experiences of many teenagers (Lovegrove 2002).

*Self-processes*

In a seven-year cohort study carried out in the USA, Prokhorov et al. (1993) reported that their sample of 2406 adolescents rated appearance as the most valued characteristic in their lives (compared with school performance, family, food, money, exercise, friends and watching TV). The authors also noted that appearance was the only one of these factors that increased in value over time.

Lovegrove (2002, Lovegrove and Rumsey 2005) designed a research programme exploring appearance concerns, and appearance-related teasing and bullying in 671 secondary school pupils. Responses to the question: 'How does your appearance affect the way you feel about yourself?' resulted in numerous examples of the close link between perceptions of appearance and feelings about the self. Forty-four per cent responded that looks confer self confidence:

> The better you look, the more confident you are around people.
>
> (Female, 14 years)

> If I look in the mirror and don't like my appearance I feel upset and angry and I don't like myself.
>
> (Male, 11 years)

> When I don't like my appearance, I don't like myself because I feel other people judge me on that. It gives me low esteem which makes it all worse.
>
> (Female, 15 years)

The first quote represents those (40 per cent) who reported that if they felt more attractive they also felt more positive about themselves.

In an attempt to unpick the links between self-esteem and evaluations of appearance, Harter (1999) asked adolescents which caused the other. She found that 60 per cent of adolescents thought that self-evaluations came first, preceding and determining self-worth. Girls taking this view reported that appearance was of more importance, that they were more preoccupied with their appearance, and that they worried more about how they looked to others. They felt worse about their appearance, had lower self-esteem and felt more depressed than the second group of teenage girls (40 per cent of

Harter's sample) who felt that self-worth determined self-perceptions of appearance. In Lovegrove's study, when asking what aspects of their appearance they disliked, 26 per cent of respondents wanted to weigh less, 15 per cent wanted better skin, and 8 per cent wanted to change the shape of their nose or ears. When asked what they liked, eyes came out top (28 per cent of the sample), followed by hair (22 per cent) and facial appearance (10 per cent). However, 18 per cent felt that had no good features at all, and 9 per cent of participants only liked the clothes they wore. Fifty-one per cent of the respondents in Lovegrove's (2002) study expected their current concerns to be specific to adolescence and young adulthood:

> I suppose I'll change. By the time I'm 25, I'll care more about my character.
>
> (Male, 14 years)

> Once I'm married, I won't feel the need to impress any more.
>
> (Female, 12 years)

> I'll always worry because now it's spots, but later it'll be a beer belly and wrinkles.
>
> (Male, 16 years)

*Responses from others*

Thompson et al. (2002) noted the compelling evidence that teasing is associated with body dissatisfaction and other forms of distress during adolescence, citing as an example a study by Fabian and Thompson (1989) who noted that teasing frequency and the degree of resulting distress were associated with higher levels of body dissatisfaction, eating disturbance, depression and lower self-esteem. Wardle and Collins (1998) used a sample of 766 12 to 16 year olds from Dublin and London, and also found teasing and body dissatisfaction to be related, with teasing from family a more important predictor than teasing at school. Garner (1997) in the *Psychology Today* survey reported that 44 per cent of women and 35 per cent of men noted that 'being teased by others' was a contributory factor in their body image. Rieves and Cash (1996) asked 111 college women which aspect of their appearance had been the target of teasing, and also asked about the perpetrators of this teasing. They found that 45 per cent had been teased about the face and head, and 36 per cent about their weight. The most frequent source of teasing was brothers (79 per cent), followed by peers (62 per cent). Thomas et al. (1998) found that fear of negative appearance evaluation is significantly correlated with body dissatisfaction and is also higher in those with a history of being teased. Crozier and Dimmock (1999) cited verbal harassment in the form of name calling and nicknames as the most prevalent form of bullying in school and reported appearance-related bullying in over 50 per cent of their sample of 45 school-age adolescents.

In Lovegrove's study, 51 per cent of adolescents reported that they feared appearance related teasing and bullying in school. However, she noted that the reported incidence levels were highest in younger teenagers (75 per cent of her sample of 11 to 14 year olds), and declined gradually up to the age of 19:

> Being thin and beautiful makes you popular. If you aren't, you get bullied like me.
>
> (Female, 12 years)

Lovegrove also noted that boys in co-educational schools were much more concerned with appearance issues than their contemporaries attending boys-only schools.

*Family influences*

In the body image literature, maternal modelling of weight loss behaviour is commonly reported by secondary school-aged girls (see for example, Tiggeman 2004). However, although research is limited, it would appear that there are considerable differences in the extent to which families are openly supportive or critical of the appearance of their offspring during adolescence. The majority of respondents in Lovegrove's study felt that their physical appearance did not exert an undue effect on their home lives. Nineteen per cent said that their family was generally positive about the way they looked, although 27 per cent of 12 year olds did say that their parents 'expected certain standards of appearance'. Active parental disapproval of the appearance of participants was reported with a frequency that increased with age, with levels peaking at 27 per cent of 17 and 18 year olds. Some found this parental disapproval distressing:

> It affects me tremendously when my mother makes bad comments.
>
> (Female, 17 years)

Twenty-nine per cent of Lovegrove's sample said they talked to their mothers when they had appearance concerns. This was more common for girls (37 per cent) than for boys (20 per cent). A further 16 per cent said they talked to both parents, with only 2 per cent approaching their fathers. Fifty-two per cent reported a preference for talking to their friends.

*Societal influences*

As with pre-teens, many adolescents are voracious consumers of the media, particularly magazines, television 'soaps' and films. Levine and Smolak (1996) found that 83 per cent of teenage girls reported spending an average of 4.3 hours each week reading magazines, with 70 per cent rating them as important sources of information about beauty and fitness. Some writers have noted that teenagers may also be particularly vulnerable to appearance messages transmitted in the media, as they have high levels of concern about the way they look and are evaluated by others (Smolak 2004). They are caught in the paradox of wanting to qualify as 'normal', yet have high levels of exposure to images that are heavily skewed towards the top end of the physical attractiveness continuum. Harter (1999) has noted first that the appearance stereotypes portrayed in the media have become more and more extreme and difficult to match, and second that magazines now frequently include computer 'enhanced' images of models in which unlikely combinations of features (for example, large breasts and slim hips), have been artificially combined and yet are presented as desirable (see Chapter 8).

*The consequences of appearance concerns for teenagers*

The potential impact of appearance-related concerns during adolescence is considerable. This is one of the many areas in need of more research, but Lovegrove's study gives a clear message about the pervasive nature of appearance concerns in secondary school pupils and the ramifications for the daily lives of the majority of her sample. Forty-four per cent felt that 'looking good' contributed significantly to their social confidence. Age increased this effect, with 18 per cent of 11 year olds making this link, rising to 78 per cent of 18 year olds. Forty per cent associated appearance with self-esteem, saying that if they felt they were looking good, they also felt good about themselves. Most of those who were unhappy with their appearance felt their social life was affected. More surprisingly, 31 per cent of participants felt their academic confidence was also affected, and claimed not to speak up in class because they feared attention being drawn to their appearance:

> No way am I speaking up when I know they're gonna laugh at my big arse.
>
> (Male, 15 years)

In addition, 20 per cent of Lovegrove's 15-year-olds sample claimed to truant from school because of their appearance, with many lacking the confidence or skill to deal with teasing effectively:

> If you go out you think people are pointing and laughing at you, so you stay home.
>
> (Female, 14 years)

> I spend my whole life trying to look thinner and prettier so that people will like me and not bully me.
>
> (Female, 13 years)

Dieting in adolescence is widespread and often restrictive. The use of smoking as an appetite suppressant is common, especially among girls. Increasing numbers of teenagers are both contemplating and undergoing cosmetic surgery (Sarwer and Crerand 2004), and Haste (2004) has reported that the desire to improve appearance and lose weight is strongly linked to the motivation to exercise, especially for girls. This author also noted that anxieties about appearance can also inhibit exercise, for example the desire not to develop bulky muscles, or self consciousness about appearing in appropriate clothing (see Chapter 2). Teenage boys engage in weight training in increasing numbers, and muscle definition and bulk are increasingly becoming a prerequisite for membership of school and local teams. There are risks associated with overexercising however. To achieve the necessary muscle mass, boys are taking protein supplements, and in some cases, anabolic steroids from a tender age (Santrock 2001). The potential side effects of these are considerable, including several that impact on appearance, such as severe acne, shrinking testicles, a reduced sperm count, premature baldness, enlarged prostate glands, an increase in breast tissue, pain or difficulty on urinating, and even a possibly increased risk of liver cancer.

### Adulthood

#### Appearance and self-perceptions

Interest in self-processes burgeoned within social and developmental psychology in the 1990s, but little was made of the role of appearance at this time. However, for appearance researchers, Harter (1999) and her colleagues stand out as beacons in this research, partly because of their attempts to impose order on the plethora of self terminologies, but also because of the attention they paid to people's assessments of their physical appearance as a component of the self-processes. Harter made a useful distinction between global and specific domains of the self. The global perspective relates to judgements of overall self-esteem and self-worth, and is more resistant to change than the separate domains. On the basis of her own research and a review of other relevant work, Harter believes that the specific domains include scholastic competence, social acceptance, physical appearance, behavioural conduct and athletic competence. Her results indicate that of all the domains, physical appearance has the strongest association with global self-worth. In work with adolescents and young adults she has reported correlations of 0.52–0.80, with a mean of 0.65 in the USA and 0.62 in other countries. The other domains achieve associations of between 0.30 and 0.48. Harter and her co-workers have concluded that at every developmental level up to and including middle age, evaluations of one's looks take precedence over other domains as the main predictors of self-worth. However, not all researchers are so convinced. Langlois et al. (2000) found only weak support for the assertion that people rated by others as attractive or unattractive have different self-views. In addition, although some studies suggest that attractive adults perceive themselves as more competent and more mentally healthy than their unattractive counterparts, the effect sizes are smaller than in research exploring the impact of a person's appearance on the perceptions and behaviours of other people.

More food for thought concerning the appearance-related components of self-perceptions has come from the body image literature. Thompson (1990) for example, defined body image in terms of three principal components. The first is *perceptual*, reflecting a person's view of his or her own physical appearance. The second is *evaluative*, comprising a person's attitudes towards his or her body. This author proposed that these attitudes consist of both a value (the degree of satisfaction or dissatisfaction with one's body) and a valance (a measure of the importance of body image to one's self-esteem). More recently, researchers have further refined the detail and measurement of the psychological importance of appearance-related beliefs and cognitions to the individual's sense of self and self-worth and the extent to which a person's thoughts and behaviours actively centre round appearance (Cash et al. 2004). For Thompson, the third component is *behavioural*, and relates to the degree to which a person's behaviours are affected by perceptions or feelings about the body.

The lack of a relationship between perceived and objective ratings of appearance has been an intriguing focus of interest for researchers in this area. Feingold's (1992) meta-analysis of attractiveness research offered evidence for the relative distinctiveness of the subjective (self-ratings) versus objective ratings of attractiveness. He found correlations of 0.24 for men and 0.25 for women, concluding that just over 6 per cent of a person's own view of appearance is explained by actual attractiveness as rated by others. Feingold found that one's own self-rating of attractiveness was significantly associated with global self-esteem, but failed to find a corresponding relationship with objective ratings.

It has also become evident that self-perceptions are a movable feast. The self is fluid and fluctuates to become closer or further away from individual and cultural ideals over both brief and longer periods of time. Some changes occur only gradually, for example those associated with ageing, but others are more dramatic. The experience of pregnancy arguably offers one of the greatest naturally occurring potential deviations from a bodily ideal during adulthood. Johnson et al. (2004) analysed interviews with six pregnant women. Rather than delight in the physical changes associated with pregnancy, the overwhelming experience of the participants was one of feeling 'fat', 'frumpy' and less physically attractive (with the exception of enjoying an increase in breast size). The experience of one participant – a woman who described herself as 'British Asian' – served to highlight the impact of custom and practice on self-perceptions and appearance concerns among different ethnic groups. This participant engaged in the Indian cultural ritual of not washing her hair for the first seven months of her pregnancy, and reported that this had a detrimental impact on how she felt she looked in comparison with other pregnant women.

Melynk and colleagues (2004) examined the fluidity of body image ratings over a period of six days. They found that those participants who had more negative body image ratings and who invested more actively in appearance-management strategies were more liable to fluctuations in body image state ratings. Langlois et al. (2000) noted that more longitudinal studies are needed to clarify the extent of stability and change. However, even these types of studies would be unlikely to capture the full complexity of short- and long-term temporal fluctuations. To complicate matters further, a person thinks or acts in relation to a number of different identities, which can be defined at an individual, small or large group level, or combinations of levels at any one time. This can be easier to conceptualize as each of us having a number of personas, which we present to the world in the context of the various settings we enter, for example in work, home or social situations. Associated with these presentations are image displays. For some identities, the detail of the self-presentation may be similar, whereas others result in greater variation. Although the external image may offer only a 'mere sliver' of who we are, other people read a whole personality into the way we present ourselves. Stereotyping by others is a well-established focus of research by social psychologists, but there is also evidence that people self-stereotype (Levine 1999): they ascribe to themselves norms and values associated with different identities as each becomes salient. There is considerable variation in the importance ascribed to appearance in these processes. Harter (1999) has pointed out that the self is both a cognitive and a social construct – two distinct, but intertwined aspects. The wider socio-cultural context will influence the content and valence attached to appearance in a person's self-representation, as will the value each individual associates with meeting cultural standards of appearance. (See Chapter 5 for a more comprehensive discussion of these issues.)

*The impact of appearance on others*

Garner (1997) described our external appearance as our personal billboard, providing others with information on which they base their first – and sometimes only – impressions. These inferences were studied extensively during the 1970s and 1980s by social psychologists (see Chapter 1). Despite the prevailing emphasis on body shape and weight in the body image literature, the face is considered by most researchers to be the body part which is the primary focus of most first encounters. Accordingly, it is the impact of facial appearance on others which has been the main interest for researchers in this area.

The majority of the many studies in this area during the 1970s and 1980s reported the pervasive benefits of a physically attractive facial appearance. Two notable meta-analyses of research in this area offered a synthesis of these studies and some interesting pointers for subsequent work. Eagly et al.

(1991) summarized 76 studies in which participants of 14 years or over inferred the attributes of people they did not know from photographs. The authors concluded that the physical attractiveness stereotype was not as strong or as general as implied by previous researchers, with effect sizes moderate at best. They noted that the process of stereotyping is affected by the type of inference participants are asked to make and that the effects were largest for indices of social competence. Intermediate effect sizes were found for ratings of adjustment and intellectual competence, and near zero effects in relation to integrity and concern for others. They concluded that the core of the physical attractiveness stereotype concerns sociability and popularity. An important additional finding was that the more information that was available in addition to stimulus photographs, the less importance was ascribed to appearance. Eagly and colleagues' findings led them to predict that looks would be less important in perceptions of friends, family and co-workers than they are for strangers.

Langlois et al. (2000) found that judges showed high levels of agreement when evaluating the attractiveness of photographs of both adults ($r = 0.90$) and children ($r = 0.85$). They were also surprised by the levels of cross-ethnic agreement ($r = 0.88$) and cross-cultural agreement (0.94). More attractive adults were thought to be better at their jobs, to have more social appeal, more interpersonal competence, and to be better adjusted. They were found to be offered more attention, a greater number of positive interactions, fewer negative interactions, and more help. Unlike Eagly, Langlois and colleagues included the variable 'familiarity with the target person' in their regression equations, but found no effect. Neither were any significant gender or age effects apparent.

They concluded that attractive adults are both judged and treated more positively than unattractive adults, even by those who know them, and that the effects of facial attractiveness are 'robust and pandemic', including initial impressions and actual interactions. Attractiveness is considered by this research group as a significant advantage for adults in many spheres of life. The authors did note that few studies had examined the presumed causal link between treatment by others and the differential behaviour exhibited by attractive and less attractive people.

*Appearance and the reciprocal nature of social interaction*

The links between the perceptions and behaviours of others and the perceptions and behaviours of a target person are difficult to unravel. Notwithstanding the complexities of the self-perception literature, research concerning the responses of others is currently fragmented into studies of impression formation, judgements made of the target person by others, and the behaviour of others towards the target person (Langlois et al. 2000). There has been little attempt to integrate these areas, and all too often the conceptual links between these areas of research are lacking.

While acknowledging some gaps in the evidence, Langlois et al. (2000) attempted to link the findings of their meta-analyses by using some explanatory aspects of socialization and social expectancy theories. These included the processes of behavioural confirmation and self-fulfilling prophecy theories which had previously been favoured as explanatory frameworks (see Bull and Rumsey (1988) and Rumsey (1997)). Langlois and her colleagues also considered the ideas developed by evolutionary theorists to be worthy of exploration.

Socialization and social expectancy theories have the advantage of being plausible and intuitively appealing. These perspectives postulate first that cultural norms and experiences influence the behaviour of both parties in an interaction, and second, that social stereotypes create their own reality. Langlois et al. (2000) concluded that there is considerable evidence that the behaviour of others is affected by appearance. They proposed that attractive people elicit expectations that are different from those lacking in attractiveness, and cited evidence in their article that these expectations are acted upon differently. There is, however, relatively little research addressing the other assumptions of these theories, namely that these processes promote differential behaviour in the target person, and the target comes to internalize these judgements, developing different behaviour patterns and views of the self. The literature on self-perception does offer some support for this explanation; however clearly, the extent to which these processes apply varies considerably from person to person. Take for example, the attentional mechanisms in social encounters. Some people appear to be highly attuned to signs of approval and disapproval from others, whereas others have a more robust self-view and are less concerned about picking up feedback of this type (Heinrichs and Hofmann 2001).

Although there is little evidence to support the mechanisms proposed by evolutionary theorists to explain the effects of physical attractiveness on the behaviour of others, the theories make interesting reading. Various evolutionary perspectives share the view that attractive faces are biological 'ornaments' signalling valuable information to others. Penton-Voak and Perrett (2000a) maintain that an attractive face acts as a kind of 'health certificate' indicating the person's value as a potential mate. Men will seek out attractive women and behave towards them more positively, as they believe they are the most likely to be fit, healthy and able to contribute 'high quality' genes to the potential joint offspring. Women, however, place a greater emphasis on 'resources' in prospective mates than on physical attractiveness in the expectation that the resourceful male can better provide for the potential offspring.

Some interesting 'twists' to appearance research are offered by evolutionary theorists, particularly in relation to judgements of physical attractiveness. High testosterone levels in males are desirable in evolutionary terms as they are thought to indicate strength and aggression. Higher levels result in a forward growth of the brow ridges, and an increase in the size of jaw bones, the lower face and cheekbones. Oestrogen levels in women and associated assumptions of fertility can be assessed by onlookers through the facial bone architecture and lip fullness. Women's judgements of men are further complicated by cyclic preferences. Penton-Voak and Perrett (2000b) claim to have established that women prefer more masculine faces in the follicular phase of the menstrual cycle and more 'feminine' male faces at other times. In addition, these choices are also affected by the type of relationship sought. There are apparently no changes in preferences across the menstrual cycle when expressing choices for a long-term partner, only when a short-term one is being contemplated. In addition, Frost (1994) found that around the time of ovulation, women prefer relatively darker male skin (also apparently a sign of masculinity).

An additional theory from the evolutionary stable is that early childhood experience and learning may influence our later attractiveness and sexual preferences in a way that is analogous to the imprinting mechanism common in birds. These mechanisms are predicted to lead people to favour potential partners with a familial resemblance. There is a little evidence of similarity and familial resemblance in partner studies (see Chapter 1), but although it is the kind of theory that might enliven a dinner conversation, currently evidence for this idea is tenuous at best.

Eagly et al. (1991) favoured implicit personality theory as a theoretical framework to explain the findings of their meta-analysis. From this perspective, stereotypes act as knowledge structures which help people make sense of the behaviour of others. Stereotypes are construed as cognitive structures whose primary components are personal attributes (personality traits) and inferential relations that specify the degree to which the attributes co-exist and co-vary (in this case, inferential relationships that link physical attractiveness and personal attributes). These 'implicit personality theories' are developed on the basis of two main inputs. First, through direct observations of the temperament and behaviour of attractive and unattractive people in one's social environment, and second, through exposure to cultural representations of attractive and unattractive people. Eagly and colleagues find this heuristic more helpful than the more blanket approach of the 'what is beautiful is good' hypothesis put forward by Dion (1973), which infers that attractiveness is strongly linked with a range of positive characteristics, as implicit personality theory helps to explain why some attributes are more strongly linked to appearance than others.

Are there actually differences in temperament and behaviour which are attributable to physical appearance? Feingold (1992) reported significant relationships between attractiveness and measures of mental health, social anxiety, popularity and sexual activity, but there were no significant relationships between attractiveness and levels of sociability, levels of internal locus of control, or levels of self-absorption. Langlois et al. (2000) have, however, pointed out that Feingold's work related in the main to the results of psychometric tests rather than observations of actual behaviour.

Langlois et al. (2000) concluded from their meta-analysis that attractive children behaved more positively and possessed more positive traits than their unattractive peers (see Chapter 1). These children were more popular, had better psychological adjustment and better academic performance indicators. The age at which these differences manifest themselves is not clear, and more research involving young children is needed. Attractive adults achieved more occupational success, were liked more by others, engaged in more dating behaviour and had more sexual experience. They were more extroverted, had more self-confidence and self-esteem, somewhat better social skills and slightly better mental health.

Despite some reservations about the methodologies employed by appearance researchers, it is clear that physical appearance has a pervasive impact on the self-perceptions and behaviour of many. Rosen and colleagues (1997) have illustrated the multifactorial nature of the impact of appearance on adjustment through their synthesis of hundreds of accounts offered by students and patients of critical events, experiences and processes in their lives. The authors developed 19 categories of factors they maintain are predictive of body image disturbance. These include cognitive processes such as the development of self-esteem and social comparison, emotional responses such as feelings of acceptance or fear of rejection and lifestyle factors such as participation in exercise, the effects of familial and peer values and attitudes, feedback from others and actual physique. These processes do not take place in a vacuum. They are influenced by a person's societal and cultural context, by life events, and also by developmental stage.

*Societal influences*

Before the advent of mass media, images of beauty were communicated through art, music and literature (Thompson et al. 2002). Freedman (1986) explored the evidence that historically, beauty ideals were romanticized and interpreted as unattainable. However, contemporary media blur the boundaries between glorified fiction and reality. Carefully manipulated images and computer merged composites of the 'best' features of more than one model are presented as realistic, appropriate standards for comparison for readers and viewers (Lakoff and Scherr 1984). Those exposed to the images have little or no notion of the massive input from professionals in their production, and certainly have precious little chance of matching the investment of time, finance or professional input necessary to achieve the 'look' portrayed (see Chapter 8).

Many researchers have noted the powerful effects of societal factors on the development and maintenance of body image disturbance in westernized societies (Thompson et al. 2002). In the 1997 *Psychology Today* survey, of the 3452 women responding, 23 per cent indicated that movie or television celebrities had influenced their body image aspirations when they were young, with 22 per cent endorsing the influence of fashion models portrayed in magazines (Garner 1997).

It takes only a cursory glance at the print media (particularly women's fashion magazines) to confirm that publishers regularly endorse unattainable images and standards. Many millions buy magazines regularly and millions more access magazines via friends, libraries, waiting rooms, hairdressers and coffee shops. Levine and Smolak (1992) reported that 68 per cent of female university students felt worse about their physical appearance after reading women's magazines. Thirty-three per cent of the sample reported that fashion advertisements made them feel less satisfied with their appearance, and 50 per cent reported that they wished they looked more like models advertising cosmetics. Ironically, the advertisements for cosmetic surgery which can be found in the classified section of the vast majority of women's and increasing numbers of men's magazines also make widespread use of all-too-perfect models portrayed through soft focus lenses. Some even depict equally good looking partners and use an exotic location as a back-drop. These advertisements imply that plastic surgery is the way to achieve similar flawless looks, together with a better life and happier future.

Garner (1997) found that 27 per cent of women and 12 per cent of men always or very often compared themselves to models in magazines, and 28 per cent of women and 19 per cent of men carefully studied the shapes of models. When respondents were stratified on body image disturbance, 43 per cent of dissatisfied women compared themselves with the shape of models. Sixty-seven per cent of extremely dissatisfied women reported that thin models made them feel insecure about their weight, and made them want to lose weight, and 45 per cent reported feeling angry or resentful in response to such exposure.

Television is a pervasive, commonly used medium for the communication of standards of attractiveness. However, the type of programme watched, rather than merely exposure is clearly important. Heinberg and Thompson (1995) showed female college students ten-minute videotapes of com-mercials with stimuli emphasizing ideals of thinness and attractiveness, or neutral, non-appearance related content. Results showed that those who viewed the tape stressing the importance of appearance reported higher levels of depression, anger, dissatisfaction with weight and overall appearance, than those viewing the other recording. However, the effects were not the same for all. Those with high levels of body image dissatisfac-tion showed increased levels of dissatisfaction, whereas those with lower body image dissatisfaction showed reductions following exposure. All parti-cipants had reductions in dissatisfaction after the neutral video. Groesz et al. (2002) concluded from a meta-analysis of studies examining body (dis)satis-faction in girls and young women after viewing idealized media images, that body image was significantly more negative after exposure, and that in some studies, levels of depression and anxiety were increased.

In relation to differences in susceptibility to media messages, Thompson et al. (2002) have discussed the likelihood that awareness and mere exposure to societal pressures may not be sufficient to explain body image disturbance, and that people vary in relation to their level of acceptance or 'buying into' the ideals promulgated by the media. Humphreys and Paxton (2004) showed 106 14- to 16-year-old boys advertisements depicting either lean, athletic and muscular bodies or non-figure adverts. Although there were no overall effects of the idealized images on the viewers, prior levels of body dissatisfaction predicted negative responses to ratings of anxiety and body shape. Higher pre-exposure levels of internalization of the idealized male image predicted negative shifts in body image and depression. Using female participants, Halliwell and Dittmar (2004) also found that internalization of sociocultural ideals was a strong predictor of body image disturbance after viewing advertisements. In their study varying the body size of the female models depicted, they found that exposure to thin (rather than average-size) models resulted in greater body-focused anxiety in women who were high on internalization of thin sociocultural ideals.

Thompson et al. (2002) have noted that more research is needed to explore the charactieristcs of those who are more successful in challenging these messages, and have also pointed out that the causal direction of media influence remains unclear. It is not yet known whether exposure is an aetiological factor in body image dissatisfaction and disturbance, or whether those with pre-existing high levels choose to expose themselves to such images at a higher rate than less distressed counterparts. Laying the blame squarely on the prevailing societal backdrop may seem tempting, but is not a sufficient explanation. The interaction between current sociocultural pressures and other factors including the influence of peers and family, cognitive processes such as internalization and social comparison tendencies must also be accounted for (see Chapter 6).

*The consequences of appearance concerns in adulthood*

In her research exploring the concerns of 300 adults, Liossi (2003) identified that appearance dissatisfaction could take the form of mild feelings of unattractiveness through to a pervasive obsession with physical appearance. From the perspective of a clinical psychologist, she noted that it was difficult to determine at which point a person's perceptions, attitudes and behaviours become problematic or pathological. She posed the currently unanswerable question of where to draw the boundary between normative discontent and pathological dissatisfaction.

Liossi also noted that the participants in her research who had high levels of appearance concerns actively attempted to control their appearance by various means, including diet, exercise and cosmetic surgery. Ogden (1992) estimated that 95 per cent of women have dieted at some stage in their lives, with about 40 per cent dieting at any one time. The proportion of men who admit to dieting is significantly less than women, yet recent reports claim that around 25 per cent of men are dieting at any one time (Prynn 2004).

Wilcox (1997) estimated that about 50 per cent of women under the age of 40 engage in some kind of exercise, and reported that body dissatisfaction was greater in women who did not exercise compared with those who were more active. Donaldson (1996) reported that 65 per cent of men said they engaged in sport specifically to improve their body shape and musculature. Fawkner's research (personal communication) suggests that body image dissatisfaction is a major motivator of risky appearance maintenance behaviours in men, including excessive exercise and the use of steroids to increase muscle mass. Fawkner has also found indications that men with high levels of body dissatisfaction may adopt riskier sexual practices than those who are more satisfied with their physical appearance (see Chapter 5).

Appearance concerns also motivate many people to spend a significant proportion of their income on cosmetics and other 'aids' marketed as appearance enhancers. In addition to the many lotions and potions which allegedly perform miracles for both sexes (such as 'reversing the signs of ageing'), underwear departments tempt women and teenage girls to buy from a bewildering array of elasticated undergarments, all of which offer the promise of 'improving' the appearance of different aspects of the body, including legs, thighs, bottoms, stomachs and breasts.

Since the 1990s, there have been significant increases in the numbers of both women and men who are motivated to improve their appearance by undergoing cosmetic surgery (see Chapter 6). Hall (1995) has noted that increasing numbers of adults are expressing their unhappiness with facial characteristics which imply ethnic membership, for example, a prominent nose or the shape of the eyes. Hari (2003) reported a 'near epidemic' in the USA of people of Jewish, Asian or black origin who want aspects of their faces altered to more closely resemble the westernized 'norms'. Worryingly, the worship of stars portrayed in the media seems to be taking on a more extreme dimension, with many candidates for plastic surgery motivated by the desire to look more like the stars. To make this task easier, two American plastic surgeons, Fleming and Mayer, compiled and published a list in 1998 of the most frequently requested features of stars and who 'owned them' (Kemp et al. 2004). In the popular MTV series *I Want a Famous Face*, contestants compete to undergo extensive surgery with the aim of looking more like their favourite celebrity.

### Older adulthood

The physical signs of ageing have been the subject of extensive comment in recent years, and few have attracted a positive press. The hair loses its colour and becomes thinner. Skin sags and becomes drier. The chin doubles, ear-lobes grow bigger and the nose broadens and lengthens. Wrinkles become progressively more pronounced. In addition, there is an accumulation of threats and changes imposed by nature during later life. Older people are more likely to have to deal with the impact of appearance-changing chronic conditions, for example, to joints, weight, posture or skin. Some may also have to employ unwelcome visible aids, including glasses and walking sticks (Tiggemann 2004). Despite these extensive changes to appearance, research exploring related concerns in this age group is currently very limited.

In one of the few studies to have compared levels of distress across the adult years, Montepare (1996) found that levels of body dissatisfaction in women aged 17–85 were consistently high. However, Harris and Carr (2001) reported lower levels of appearance concerns in older adults. For women, the prevalence of higher levels of concern was greatest in the sample aged 18–30 years, affecting 69 per cent of participants. This level declined slightly to 60 per cent of respondents in the 51–60-year-old group. The lowest levels of concern were in the 61 years and over grouping (33 per cent). For men, the highest levels of concern were also in those aged 18–21 years (56 per cent of participants), falling progressively to a figure of 24 per cent in the 51–60 group, and 21 per cent in the participants who were 61 years and over.

Some other commentators have also suggested that the importance attached to outward appearance appears to decrease with age. Tiggeman (2004) noted that relationships between body dissatisfaction and self-esteem appeared to be weaker in samples of people aged 50–65 than they were in younger (20–35 years) and in middle-aged samples (35–50 years), although the mechanisms of this effect are unclear and remain speculative at present. It may be that in some cases the emphasis of concern may shift to the more functional aspects of appearance (for example, the functioning of eyes, or perhaps that self-perceptions of appearance have less impact on perceptions of identity and global self-esteem than previously). Grogan (1999) suggested that with advancing age people may shift their focus of comparison to age-appropriate peers more than to media ideals, and that they become more realistic about what is achievable. Although Tiggemann (2004) noted that older adults continue to use appearance management strategies, it may be that they become concerned with the more easily controllable aspects of grooming – including hair, clothes and jewellery – than with matching ideals portrayed in the media. This is illustrated by the words of a 60-year-old female participant in a qualitative interview study reported by Halliwell and Dittmar (2003):

> You don't have to be this glamorous person as you get older, although you still want to look nice.

Tiggemann added the hopeful notion that perhaps by a later stage in life, adults have come to appreciate diversity in appearance. As a result of these various processes, the otherwise socially undesirable and largely uncontrollable age-related body changes may be associated with less distress than would otherwise be the case. Tunalcy et al. (1999) completed in-depth interviews with 12 British women aged 63–75. Although all the participants said they would prefer to have a slimmer appearance, they had reduced their feelings of personal responsibility and guilt for weight gain by attributing this to the unavoidable biological consequences of ageing. The women appeared more resistant to sociocultural ideals of beauty, felt there was less pressure for them to look physically attractive to their partners and to others and that, with advancing age, it was acceptable to worry less about their looks.

Appearance concerns in relation to life phase transitions involve a complex combination of biological, social and psychological changes. In addition, there is considerable individual variation within each developmental stage. Longitudinal research is needed to unpick these processes, as currently, research relies on cross-sectional studies of cohorts in age groups rather than to changes to individuals across the lifespan.

## Conclusion

Appearance concerns are pervasive across the lifespan in western societies to the extent that discontent is considered by many researchers and social commentators to be normative. The concerns and distress experienced by those most affected leads them to engage in a variety of activities across the lifespan. Some of these behaviours can be considered beneficial, for example, moderate levels of exercise. Others however, are of more concern, including restrictive or unhealthy diets, excessive exercise and smoking for weight control. The increasing prevalence of risky behaviours in younger age groups is of particular concern. However, this current 'epidemic' of appearance concerns has been largely ignored by health psychologists and health promoters.

## Chapter summary

◆ The number of people experiencing high levels of appearance concern are reaching epidemic proportions in westernized societies. Rodin et al. (1985) have coined the term 'normative discontent' to describe this phenomenon;
◆ Research on appearance concerns has focused predominantly on the impact of physical appearance on self-perception; and the impact of appearance on the behaviour of others;
◆ A complex range of factors contribute to the development and maintenance of appearance concerns from early childhood onwards. These include cognitive processes; emotional responses; family environment; lifestyle factors; peer values; the responses of others; the social cultural context; actual physical appearance and developmental stage.

## Discussion points

♦ Is 'normative discontent' with appearance an inherent part of the human experience, or is it a product of our times?
♦ How might the responses of others and appearance-related self-perceptions influence each other?
♦ What have been the most powerful influences on the way you feel about your own appearance?
♦ To what extent do appearance issues influence your health behaviours?

## Further reading

Grogan, S. (1999) *Body Image: Understanding Body Dissatisfaction in Men, Women and Children*. London: Routledge.
Langlois, J.H., Kalakanis, L., Rubenstein, A.J., Larson, A., Hallam, M. and Smoot, M. (2000) Maxims or myths of beauty? A meta-analytic and theoretical review. *Psychological Bulletin*, 126: 390–423.
Thompson, J.K., Heinberg, L.J., Altabe, M. and Tantleff-Dunn, S. (1999) *Exacting Beauty: Theory, Assessment and Treatment of Body Image Disturbance*. Washington, DC: American Psychological Association.

# Psychological difficulties associated with visible difference

Whether first evident at birth, or acquired later in life, a visible difference can have a profound impact upon the affected person. MacGregor (1979) argued that a visible difference comprises a 'social disability', since in addition to impacting on the thoughts, feelings and behaviours of those affected, it is also likely to influence the behaviour of other people. However, recent research suggests that the extent to which a visible difference results in social disability involves a complex interplay of social and individual factors (Rumsey and Harcourt 2004; Thompson and Kent 2001).

## Defining what is and is not a disfigurement

Drawing the boundary around what does and does not constitute a disfigurement is far from straightforward. The perspective of the affected person may differ from that of others who observe the disfigurement, and the views of both parties will be affected by their past experience, attitudes, values and by the prevailing sociocultural environment. Attempts to measure appearance objectively have been largely unsuccessful (Roberts-Harry 1997), and there is no defined range of what is 'normal' and 'abnormal' – for example, at what point, if at all, does a large nose constitute a disfigurement (Harris 1997)? A definition adopted by several researchers is that a disfigurement is 'a difference from a culturally defined norm which is visible to others'. The significance of including 'visibility to others' is first to exclude body dysmorphic disorder in which the difference is imagined or grossly exaggerated by the affected person (Veale 2004), and second, as a result of its visibility, that the difference has the potential to affect interactions with others.

## The causes of visible difference

The UK-based charity *Changing Faces* estimates that approximately one in seven people have some kind of visible difference. However, these estimates are based on 1988 UK population census figures, and are vague at best. Visible differences result from a surprisingly wide variety of congenital anomalies, from chronic diseases such as arthritis, as a consequence of stroke, in the aftermath of injury or as the result of surgical intervention. Consequently, the exact figures are unknown, but current estimates are likely to be conservative. Using the prevalence of skin conditions as just one indicator, it is estimated that 15–20 per cent of consultations in primary care in the UK concern a dermatological disorder. Most people over the age of 65 suffer from two or more dermatological conditions worthy of medical attention, many of which are visible to others (Kligman 1989). Some form of acne affects 95 per cent of 16-year-old girls and 83 per cent of boys (Kellett 2002), with about 20 per cent of those affected seeking treatment from the health services.

### *Congenital disfigurements*

Some types of conditions causing visible differences are fully manifested at birth (for example, a cleft of the lip), whereas others become more evident over time (for example, neurofibromatosis). Harris (1997) proposed that the classification of a 'congenital disfigurement' should be those that exist 'pre-memory', that is to say that the person has no memory of life without the impairment.

Head and neck malformations are the most common visible birth 'defects'. A cleft (or gap) in the lip and/or palate occurs in approximately 1 in every 800 births, and can manifest on one (unilateral) or both (bilateral) sides of the midline of the face. Other less common anomalies result from the failure of the face to develop fully, as in the absence of an ear, the underdevelopment of cheek and jaw bones (as in Treacher-Collins syndrome), or the early fusion of the cranial bones (as in Cruzon's and Apert's syndromes). Most facial anomalies are not associated with impairments in brain function. However, there are some syndromes which involve a combination of physical features and brain impairments associated with learning difficulties (as in Down's syndrome).

Harris (1997) has summarized the anomalies which are associated with the delayed maturation of blood vessels (cutaneous haemangiamata), vascular malformations (birthmarks), or the failure of a limb to develop. Webbing ('syndactyly') refers to the failure of fingers or toes to separate fully, whereas in polydactyly an extra digit is present on the hand or foot.

*Acquired disfigurements*

These include visible differences caused by trauma (such as road traffic accidents, burns, dog bites); surgical intervention (scarring and loss of contour following the excision of tumours and surrounding tissue, the effects of chemotherapy and radiotherapy, the aftermath of cosmetic surgery); disease (for example, acne and subsequent scarring); genetic predispositions to differences that manifest in later life (vitiligo) or the absence of normal developmental processes (as in the under or asymmetric development of breasts).

## What difficulties are associated with visible difference?

The impact of disfigurement on those affected has been studied by researchers with a variety of academic backgrounds. A retrospective review is provided in Chapter 1. Sociocultural perspectives have emphasized how people's definitions and responses to disfigurement are influenced by the prevailing societal context, whereas psychological perspectives have focused on the self-perceptions, cognitions and behaviours of those affected, and ways in which a visible difference influences the cognitions and behaviours of others. The research has been amplified by several moving and very lucid personal accounts of those affected (Grealy 1994; Partridge 1990).

A detailed understanding of the appearance concerns in people with congenital or acquired conditions which cause visible differences is complicated by the need to take account of the many different types and body sites, the variability in severity and visibility, developmental stage and the numerous personal, social and situational characteristics which might affect self-perceptions and adjustment (Rumsey 2002b; see also Chapter 2). However, despite the complexity of variables involved, and the different perspectives of the researchers and writers in this area, there is a remarkable consensus concerning the 'headline' problems and difficulties. This review will first consider the challenges posed at various developmental stages, and will then explore the difficulties reported by adults in more detail. These can be roughly grouped into the experience of negative emotions such as anxiety and depression, detrimental effects on self-perceptions and self-evaluations and difficulties linked to encounters with others, together with associated emotions and behaviours such as social anxiety and social avoidance. In recent years, researchers have turned their attention to lessons that might be learned from those who adjust positively to disfigurements. Chapter 5 includes a consideration of this burgeoning area of research.

*Issues related to developmental stages*

Most of the research looking at the impact of developmental stages and adjustment to conditions resulting in visible differences have focused on the birth, childhood and adolescence of people born with a cleft lip and palate. The reasons for this are twofold. First, the fact that a cleft is the most common potentially disfiguring congenital anomaly and second, the existence of a research-active community of clinical psychologists working in this field who have underpinned their work with high-quality research. Those interested in the detail of this research are referred to an excellent review by Endriga and Kapp-Simon (1999). This review suggests that many children with craniofacial anomalies (predominantly clefts) develop in age-appropriate ways, without significant psychological problems. However, in the region of 30–40 per cent experience difficulties which are considered significant enough to be of clinical concern. These difficulties focus on combinations of shyness, social withdrawal, deficiencies in social competence, behavioural difficulties (such as disobedience or impulsivity) or impairments in cognitive functioning.

*The diagnosis of a visible congenital anomaly*

Recent advances in antenatal screening now mean that increasing numbers of parents are receiving a diagnosis of a potentially disfiguring condition before birth. In an unpublished undergraduate thesis, Farrimond and Morris (2004) estimated that currently, 20 per cent of cleft lips are identified pre-natally, and a limited number of studies have addressed the impact of this early news. Matthews et al. (1998) found in a postal survey that the majority of parents felt prenatal diagnosis had made adjustment easier at birth, and they valued the opportunity they had been given to meet with and speak to members of the cleft team prior to the birth. Most felt that the disadvantage of stress and anxiety during pregnancy was outweighed by the ability to prepare and gain relevant knowledge. Davalbhakta and Hall (2000) found 85 per cent of parents felt that a prenatal diagnosis had prepared them psychologically for the birth and 92 per cent were satisfied with the information they had been given after the diagnosis.

However, prenatal diagnosis is not without its difficulties. In most cases the scan cannot identify the extent of the cleft in the lip nor whether there are associated anomalies, such as a cleft in the palate, or a syndrome involving neurological or other impairments. Parents may imagine the worst. Farrimond's qualitative study of interviews with eight sets of parents of babies born with prenatal or postnatal diagnosis confirmed that irrespective of the timing, the discovery that the baby had a cleft was a point of crisis for all parents. Prenatal diagnosis was perceived as less of a clear-cut advantage than previous research had suggested. The additional stress during pregnancy was perceived as a major disadvantage, and parents were sometimes given conflicting information and advice from professionals prior to the birth. Some were shown photographs depicting a range of clefts and were left fearing the worst for their own infant. This response was heightened for those who had sought information about clefting from the Internet, some of which was distressing and unhelpful ('It was all doom and gloom'). Despite the drawbacks, all parents reported that prenatal diagnosis was helpful in preparing for the appearance of the baby at birth and for dealing with early feeding difficulties (a cleft can compromise the ability of the infant to suck). Most felt that on balance, it was better to know rather than to become aware of the cleft for the first time at the birth. Interestingly, however, not all the parents who were unprepared for their baby's cleft at birth felt that it would have been in their best interests to have known about the existence of the impairment beforehand.

For parents without a prenatal diagnosis, the birth of a baby with a visible congenital anomaly often comprises a major shock and disappointment (Bradbury and Hewison 1994; Farrimond and Morris 2004). The visible difference is likely to overshadow the other normal aspects of the baby, though some parents still experience a degree of elation at the safe arrival of the infant. In Farrimond's study, parents recounted a variety of negative emotional responses including disbelief, denial, anger, guilt and tearfulness. Many wanted to understand why the impairment had occurred and in particular, to explore the possibility of any personal responsibility for the cleft. Some questioned their capacity to love the infant and also their competence to cope with the initial feeding difficulties and the subsequent treatment regime. These findings concur with previous research. Endriga and Kapp-Simon (1999) reported that stress, confusion and emotional distress follow the birth or prenatal diagnosis of an infant with a cleft, in response to the multiple needs of the infant and to the ensuing treatment. Parents fear there may be additional hidden impairments, for example cognitive difficulties. They are often disappointed that breast feeding is not an option, and quickly realize that even bottle feeding will be a lengthy and stressful process at first. In Farrimond's study, these responses were relatively short lived. After the first few weeks parents reported that they had stopped noticing the cleft. So much so, that many felt ambivalent about the subsequent surgery to repair the cleft. Parents reported feelings of trauma and guilt that the surgery was taking place, as they had grown accustomed to the appearance of the cleft and didn't want the baby's appearance to change.

The reactions of health care professionals to the diagnosis and birth of the infant have a powerful impact on parents. Many report that the detail of the vivid and emotional memory of the diagnosis and/or birth of an infant with a previously undiagnosed cleft stays with them for life. Although research evidence is lacking, a calm acceptance of the existence of the cleft, a focus on the infant's other positive attributes and a brief outline of the efficacy of available treatment is helpful. Currently, whether or not the parents experience effective support is still somewhat of a lottery. There is a

need for more comprehensive training for health care p
how best to support parents at this stressful time.

The anticipated and actual reactions of family and frier
on the list of important factors in adjusting to the disfi
parents in Farrimond's study spoke of their concerns a
of others and their worries about the baby being acce
family members. They also talked of the difficulties of witnessing the shock
and disappointment of relatives when first seeing the infant, and of fears
(both real and imagined) about handling the reactions of strangers. Social
isolation can be a by-product of fear relating to the possible reactions of
others especially in the weeks and months before the surgical closure of the
cleft.

The main determinants of secure attachment are thought to be the sensitivity and responsiveness of the primary care giver to the infant (Crittenden
and Ainsworth 1989). It has been suggested that mothers may hold a baby
with a visible difference less often and that they may be less responsive to the
expressions and needs of their infants. Field and Vega-Lahr (1984) reported
that mothers of children with a craniofacial anomaly (CFA) were less active
during interactions with children at 3 months of age than mothers of
infants without a visible difference. Barden et al. (1989) examined mother–
infant interactions for babies with craniofacial differences and declared
them to be less nurturant than those where these differences were absent. In
addition to reducing attractiveness, a facial difference may affect the expressiveness of the infant. Speltz et al. (1994) reported that infants with cleft lip
and palate were less clear in their communication signals than non-cleft
infants, and also that mothers showed less responsive and sensitive behaviour
towards their offspring. Speltz and his co-authors did however report that by
the end of the first year of life, normal patterns of mother–infant behaviour
had been established. More recent studies have found few if any differences
in attachment behaviours, and researchers have concluded that although
these processes may pertain for a minority of mother–child dyads, the
majority form secure attachments and accept the disfigurement after the
initial shock has passed.

### The development of the self-concept in childhood

The impact of disfigurement on the self-concept of children has been a focus
of concern for researchers for a number of years. Early findings suggested
that the effects were predominantly negative, but more recent findings are
mixed, with several studies reporting similar self-perceptions between
groups of children with and without visible differences. In their review of
the literature relating to CFAs, Endriga and Kapp-Simon (1999) attribute
the mixed findings to problems of definition and associated measurement
issues. However, several writers have signed up to the view that positive self-
perceptions are an important correlate of higher self-esteem (Pope and

ard 1997), and that a disfigurement puts children 'at risk' for less favourable self-perceptions and self-esteem.

### Social interactions and behavioural difficulties in childhood

There is evidence that some children with unusual faces may experience
more social difficulties than their peers. Children make friendship choices
from an early age, and some research suggests that a visible difference can
affect the development of friendships. Kapp-Simon and McGuire (1997)
reported that children with facial differences both initiate and receive fewer
social approaches than those without differences. Some of those affected
have reported smaller peer groups and the desire for more friends. Endriga
and Kapp-Simon (1999) have suggested that they may engage in social
withdrawal in order to minimize the possibility of peer rejection, and that
curtailing a social network is one way of coping with the uncertainties
inherent for them in social interaction. Pope and Ward (1997) reported that
greater dissatisfaction with appearance was related to a variety of negative
symptoms in pre-adolescents, including more loneliness, fewer close friends,
social withdrawal and issues with peer relationships.

Krueckeberg et al. (1993) reported that 31 per cent of their sample of
children aged 6 to 9 were rated by teachers or parents as exhibiting
behavioural difficulties. Speltz et al. (1993) found similar levels of difficulties
in a sample of 5 to 7 year olds, with 18 per cent having clinically significant
scores. Kapp-Simon and Dawson (1998) reported cross-sectional data
on more than 300 children aged 4 to 18. Twenty per cent had clinically
significant behavioural problem scores compared to 10 per cent in a comparison group without craniofacial differences such as a cleft. Richman and
Millard (1997) have contributed a rare longitudinal study to the literature.
Their yearly assessments of more than 40 children with cleft lip and/or
palate showed gender differences in both 'internalizing' problems (such as
shyness and depression) and in 'externalizing' (for example, engaging in
antisocial or disruptive behaviour). Boys aged 4 to 12 had higher levels of
internalizing problems at all ages. In addition, boys aged 6 to 7 were higher
on externalizing problems when compared to a non-cleft group. However,
the same group scored lower than the comparison group on externalizing
problems when assessed at 11 and 12 years. Internalizing difficulties
emerged later for girls (7–12 years), and only the 12 year olds have been
reported as having higher externalizing problems than their non-cleft
peers.

### Responses from others

Reports of teasing, ridicule by others and appearance related bullying are
distressingly common from children with visible differences. Adachi et al.
(2003) found that 90 per cent of their sample of 20 women with craniofacial

differences reported teasing at school, compared with 10 per cent of their matched control sample without these facial differences.

Some researchers have explored judgements of unusual visual and vocal characteristics. Blood and Hyman (1977, reported in Endriga and Kapp-Simon 1999) reported that children gave less favourable ratings of hypernasal speakers (which is typical of some children with repaired clefts), and Tobiasen and Hiebert (1993) reported less favourable ratings in response to photographs of children with clefts. As with studies showing preferences for photos of physically attractive children compared with less attractive peers, the ecological validity of both these studies is questionable (see Chapters 1 and 2), and the impact of appearance is clearly moderated by other variables including the background attractiveness of the child in question and levels of social competence. However, these and other studies indicate that an unusual physical appearance can combine with other factors to contribute to social isolation.

### Treatment issues

Throughout childhood, treatment issues may continue to contribute to the stress of having a visible difference for all family members. For those with congenital differences, treatment will be planned well in advance. Regular check ups will remind the child and family that they have a 'difference', and the spectre of treatment may loom throughout childhood and adolescence. This treatment will often involve hospitalization and the stress of surgery. The anticipated outcomes of treatment may be over-optimistic. Some children and teenagers may expect the impossible, that is to say a completely 'normal' post-operative face, and will inevitably be disappointed with the surgical result. Alternatively, parents and children may be anxious about the effects of changes to an appearance to which they have become used to.

### Adolescence

A visible difference is thought by many researchers to cause or exacerbate existing issues relating to self-consciousness and self-esteem in adolescence. In relation to acne, disparaging lay theories about the cause of spots (lack of cleanliness, repressed anger, poor diet and so on) can contribute to self-consciousness and embarrassment about appearance. Kellett (2002) concluded that acne can be a major challenge to the self-image and group fit of adolescents, often at a crucial time in physical, psychological and sexual development. Worryingly, Cotterill and Cunliffe (1997) reported high levels of suicide ideation in adolescents with severe acne and active suicide wishes in 6 per cent of their sample of teenagers with psoriasis.

Love et al. (1987) reported a negative impact of post-burn scarring on peer relationships and social confidence in teenagers. In the Turner et al.

study (1997) of 15 and 20 year olds affected by a cleft, 60 per cent of teenagers reported being teased about their condition, with 25 per cent reporting that this teasing worried them 'a lot'. Seventy-three per cent of the sample felt their self-confidence had been very much affected by their cleft and all participants described some degree of difficulty in initiating conversations with strangers.

Appearances matter in the dating game, and for those with a visible difference, there may be a worry that an unusual appearance will be disadvantageous, resulting in a lack of confidence over making the initial moves. Kapp-Simon and McGuire (1997) used a standardized observation method to measure social interaction patterns in adolescents with and without craniofacial differences during school lunch breaks. Participants with craniofacial conditions engaged in fewer extended conversations than their comparison peers. They initiated and received fewer social approaches than those without facial differences. The authors also judged that the strategies for engaging with their peers were more tentative and less effective that those without craniofacial differences.

Although the expectation was that adolescence might be particularly challenging for those affected by clefts, in unpublished data, Emerson and Rumsey (2004) found that their sample of more than 100 cleft affected 15 year olds were equally satisfied with both their physical appearance and their friendships as were their non-affected peers. Those with a cleft rated their families as more supportive, and for both groups, satisfaction with facial appearance was positively related to family understanding.

The visible effects of treatment for cancer (including hair loss, weight changes and surgical scarring) have been shown to have a negative impact on body image when measured using standardized scales (see for example, Pendley et al. 1997). In a recent qualitative interview study involving adolescents who had experienced treatment for cancer, Wallace (2004) found appearance concerns and body image issues were an important part of the illness process. Hair loss was particularly distressing, with several participants claiming this was the worst part of treatment:

> And I was like, 'oh no, not my hair!' I wasn't worried about the treatment, I just sat there thinking, 'not my hair'.

> I wasn't really worried about anything apart from the fact that I was going to lose my hair . . . I don't like being ill. I don't like being sick or anything like that, but that side didn't seem to seem as important as the fact that I was going to lose my hair.

Appearance changes also restricted social activity and resulted in social anxiety:

> I tended not to go out with my friends in the evenings, just went to the cinema and stuff, didn't go to town with them.

I used to hang round with, like friends, but I thought . . . what they gonna say? How are they going to take it, they're not going to want to talk to me, they'll think I'm a freak or something.

Interestingly, several of Wallace's participants viewed their appearance differently after the experience of treatment and several felt it was less important than before:

Well, the way I look now, I just think . . . looks aren't everything. 'Cos I remember when I had no hair, and I was really skinny . . . I felt a freak really, but then I just thought about it and well, if people can't accept you for who you are, not what you look like, then it ain't worth it. My view to life really is, don't worry about your looks, it ain't worth it.

Others lost their fear of being 'different':

I suppose in my appearance I'm not afraid to be different anymore, you know I . . . I never used, before I used to be quite, you know, jeans, t-shirt girl, you know, just normal. Now I'd go out and buy you know, something whacky, if I liked it, I'd buy it, you know, who cares, you know?

In addition to some interesting cognitive shifts brought about by changes to appearance, researchers may wish in future to grapple with whether the heightened adolescent sensitivity to outward appearance may increase their empathy with the difficulties experienced by people with visible differences. Can we take advantage of the fact that adolescence is a life stage during which many of the problems commonly associated with visible differences are also being experienced by a significant proportion of the general population? Initial research evaluating school-based interventions to tackle appearance related teasing and bullying (Lovegrove and Rumsey 2005; see also Chapter 7) are promising.

*Treatment issues in adolescence*

Some adolescents experience difficulty in relation to involvement with decision making, especially around deciding whether to accept or decline treatment and feeling able to voice their views in consultations with health care professionals. Kapp-Simon (1995) has provided examples of the conflict that can occur between the agendas of the adolescent patient, parents and care providers. The adolescent's view could for example, be: 'I'm satisfied with the way I look, and I don't want any further treatment now', the parents' view may be: 'the doctor knows best, and we should do what s/he recommends'. Additionally, the health care providers may either advertently or inadvertently favour a particular agenda 'the optimum time for this treatment is now'. Adolescents may find hospital visits uncomfortable and may experience additional embarrassment both from feeling 'on show' in waiting areas and a 'visible specimen' in consulting rooms (Bradbury and Middleton 1997; see also Chapter 7).

*Parenting style and family issues*

A visible difference can complicate the task of parenting in a number of ways. Parents may experience difficulties in resolving their feelings about the birth of an infant with a visible difference, or in dealing with the circumstances relating to an injury to their child which results in disfigurement (see the later section on burns). As the child becomes aware of the difference, parents may avoid open discussion for fear of upsetting their offspring; however, failing to acknowledge and discuss the difference may increase the child's feeling of isolation (Bradbury 1997). The affected child or adolescent may also avoid discussing their appearance or associated problems such as teasing or bullying for fear of upsetting the parents:

> She put this barrier up to all that loved and cared for her . . . We as parents were very worried and upset to find out, years later, how much she had been bullied at school and for how long.
> (parents of Lisa, born with a facial palsy, cited in
> Lansdown et al. 1997: 66)

It is easy to understand why and how parents may come to adopt a over-protective parenting style with children affected by a visible difference (Bradbury 1997). However, the consensus view from clinicians in the area is that a more adaptive parenting style is to encourage independence and autonomy as far as possible.

An additional burden is created for many parents in the form of treatment visits. These are likely to involve taking time off work, absence from home and other family members, and additional expense. The financial burden for those without state funding or insurance cover can be punitive.

There may be effects on siblings throughout childhood and adolescence. As with physical impairments or learning difficulties, the sibling may be discriminated against socially because of their association with a visibly different child. Parents may be distracted or absent for long periods of time because of consultations and the hospitalization of the affected family member. Mothers, fathers and the marital relationship will be subjected to additional strain by worries about the affected offspring and by treatment decisions. The siblings may be reluctant to add to the burden by expressing concerns, as their problems seem relatively minor in comparison (Walters 1997).

The complex and sometimes contradictory findings summarized in this section highlight the fact that there is much more to be learned about the impact of visible difference in adolescence and we look forward to the results of ongoing research.

*Adulthood*

The difficulties experienced by people with visible differences in adulthood focus predominantly on difficulties in social encounters with others, and in relation to negative self-perceptions and emotions.

*Negative emotions*

A consistent finding in studies using standardized measures of adjustment and wellbeing is that a significant proportion of those affected have raised levels of generalized anxiety. As an illustration, in a recent study of 650 outpatients with a range of conditions resulting in visible differences, a striking 48 per cent had 'borderline case' or 'case' levels of anxiety using the Hospital Anxiety and Depression scale (Rumsey et al. 2004). There were no significant differences between patient groups when classified by condition. Similarly, researchers have found patients with skin disorders to have elevated levels of anxiety compared to normative levels. Thompson, Kent and Smith (2002) have noted a high prevalence of anxiety in people with vitiligo, and Jowett and Ryan (1985) reported that 61 per cent of their sample of 100 outpatients with a variety of skin disorders displayed symptoms of anxiety.

The incidence of significant levels of depression is generally lower than for anxiety. In the Rumsey et al. (2004) study, 27.5 per cent of the sample reported borderline case or case levels of depression. Jowett and Ryan (1985) found that a third of participants in their interview study of dermatology outpatients felt that their skin condition had significantly affected their emotional health, and reported symptoms of depression. Although depression may not constitute a headline issue for the majority, clinicians should assess their patient population carefully. Disturbingly, Herskind et al. (1993) reported a doubled suicide rate among Danish adults with clefts. Rapp et al. (1997) reported that 25 per cent of respondents to a survey of 317 people with psoriasis had considered suicide because of their condition. At the time of the survey 8 per cent thought that their life was not worth living.

*Views of the self and self-esteem*

The constructs of self-esteem, self-concept and body image continue to generate widespread debate in relation to their origins, measurement and definition. Despite the lack of consensus concerning the fine detail, there is an agreement in the literature that people with visible differences often report negative self-perceptions and unfavourable levels of self-esteem in response to their own feelings and the reactions of others to their appearance.

Van der Donk et al. (1994) reported that 75 per cent of their sample of women with alopecia (hair loss) had poor self-esteem. Moss and Carr (2004) found that variation in psychological adjustment to conditions resulting in altered appearance is related to the level of importance attached by people to their appearance, and the number of aspects of the self-system that are affected by the appearance construct. They found evidence in their sample of 70 people with visible differences that poor adjustment was related to a greater weight being attached to self-perceptions of appearance and a stronger relationship between these appearance evaluations and self-esteem. Appearance evaluations were also found to be more central in the self-system for poor adjusters, in that these were considered relevant to more aspects of the self than for good adjusters. Moss and Carr argued that when appearance evaluations are particularly dominant they are more likely to be brought to mind and used to interpret ambiguous experiences. They offer the example of a stranger who looks or stares at the affected person. If that person evaluates his or her appearance negatively, and if appearance is a sufficiently important construct to be readily available as a reference point from which to interpret this behaviour, it will be more likely that the stare will be interpreted as a negative response to the disfigurement. Similarly, if appearance plays a dominant part in the self-concept, and if the appearance is judged to be inadequate, then this will have a greater impact on overall levels of self-esteem than if a greater number of other aspects are valued (see Chapters 2 and 5).

For those with later onset disfigurement, a common report is feelings of loss of the former identity. This is a particularly frequent experience for those who undergo trauma or surgery. The inability to recognize the self or an enforced change to the appearance we are accustomed to presenting to the world, represents a profound disruption to a person's self-concept. Some writers (for example, Bradbury 1997) have talked of a process of grieving akin to a bereavement response, including elements of denial, anger, distress, anxiety and depression, followed by a gradual process of adaptation. The feelings of loss of identity that remained a year after sustaining serious burns have been eloquently described by Kwasi Afari-Mintu:

> The old Kwasi is there, somewhere at the core, but it is not possible for me to get back to him. Sometimes, when my friends come round – friends I had before the fire – I forget the scars on my hands and I don't see my face . . . Once I was a very, very confident person . . . Now I am sad; my new personality has made me sad . . . So you see what this fire has done? It's taken something of my Africanness away. How would you compensate for that?
>
> (Lansdown et al. 1997: 59)

*Anticipating negative evaluations by others*

Reports of negative emotions resulting from anxiety and fear about the possible responses of others to a visible difference are common. In the

Rumsey et al. study (2004) of outpatients seeking treatment for a range of visible conditions and injuries, mean levels of social anxiety and social avoidance were significantly raised compared with published norms (Carr et al. 2000). Levels of social distress were significantly correlated with levels of both anxiety and depression. Sixty-three per cent of the sample reported that their condition caused them to avoid some social situations, including meeting new people, places in which they felt highly visible to strangers including communal changing rooms and public swimming pools, public speaking of any kind and situations in which they might be photographed or videoed.

Leary et al. (1998) asked patients with psoriasis to complete the Brief Fear of Negative Evaluation Scale (FNE). They found an interaction between these scores and subjective distress. For patients with low FNE, the severity of the disfigurement had relatively little effect on perceptions of stigmatization, frequency of negative reactions by others, subjective distress, and interpersonal discomfort. However, the impact of severity increased as levels of FNE increased, so most distress was experienced by those whose condition was the most severe and who scored highest on the FNE, in other words, the impact of the disfigurement and its severity were moderated by the extent to which respondents were concerned with negative evaluations by others.

Miles (2002) has reported that the physical manifestations of psoriasis (flaking scaly skin and skin redness) are associated with higher levels of fear of negative evaluation by others and avoidance of social situations, including exposing the body in public places. Fortune et al. (1998) concluded that the psychosocial difficulties experienced by those with psoriasis were frequently related to high levels of anticipated anxiety about the reactions of others to their condition. Similarly, Jowett and Ryan (1985) reported that 70 per cent of their sample of 100 people with acne, psoriasis or eczema reported experiencing shame or embarrassment about the appearance of their condition, and 40 per cent said their social life had been affected. Ginsburg and Link (1989) reported people with psoriasis felt flawed, and experienced shame and secretiveness in relation to other people.

*Concepts of shame and stigma*

There are variable levels of enthusiasm for the usefulness of concepts of 'stigma' and 'shame' among researchers in this field. Gilbert (2002) described shame as the response resulting from an awareness that one has lost status and is devalued by others. Negative views about the self are defined as 'internal shame'. Coughlan and Clarke (2002) offer the example of someone who feels unattractive and worthless following a burn injury. The perception that other people view a person as unattractive and discredited is defined as 'external shame'. MacGregor (1990) in her seminal writings felt that shame was a central construct in understanding the impact of facial disfigurement: '[shame is] a predominant feeling associated with facial deviance and is central to the problem [experienced]' (p. 252, cited by Kent and Thompson 2002). More recently, an edited book on body shame (Gilbert and Miles 2002) has included contributions relating to disfigurement and shame (Kent and Thompson 2002), and more specifically shame resulting from psoriasis (Miles 2002), acne (Kellett 2002) and burns (Coughlan and Clarke 2002). The tone of the collection is that shame underpins many appearance-related psychological difficulties.

The current disagreements between researchers about the utility of this construct relate predominantly to semantics and the degree of centrality that shame occupies in the experience of visible difference. For us, shame implies humiliation, and although both internal and external shame may sometimes be a component of the experiences of those affected, we feel that the extent to which it is accurate or helpful to view shame and humiliation as central to their experiences is debatable.

Several writers have argued that people with disfigurements are also stigmatized persons (Goffman 1963; Hughes 1998; MacGregor 1990; Newell 2000b). This assertion has a certain logic when one considers that stigmata were originally marks which were deliberately inflicted on slaves to indicate their lowly position in society. Goffman, whose book *Stigma* (1963) is widely quoted by writers of this persuasion, defined stigma as implying 'something unusual or bad about the moral status of the signifier' and maintained that stigmatized people were disqualified from full social acceptance. His work explored the way in which society labels individuals or groups as deviant − including criminals, those stigmatized by membership of a particular religion or culture, and those with disabilities. Once again, we feel uneasy with the blanket application of the term to the experience of visible difference. People with disfigurements may be 'marked out' as different. They may as a result engender uncertainty and avoidance by others. But although specific experiences undoubtedly feel stigmatizing, the generalization that people with disfigurements are stigmatized, or that the majority of their experiences are necessarily stigmatizing is once again unhelpful.

*Encounters with others*

A visible difference can affect social interaction in many ways that diminish perceptions of control over encounters with others. The difficulties most frequently reported by people with visible differences relate to encounters with strangers, meeting new people and making new friends (Robinson 1997). The dislike of feeling in some way different, and the desire to achieve a state of 'normalcy' by looking unremarkable (described as 'passing' by Goffman) is strong among many people with a visible difference. Reports of staring, audible comments, unsolicited questions about the disfigurement and avoidant behaviour by members of the general public are common (Rumsey 2002b). Rather than be the object of unwanted attention, people with visible differences often yearn for privacy and anonymity − the kind of 'civil inattention' that most of us enjoy (MacGregor 1974). Jane Richardson, in talking about the experience of having severe acne, wrote that 'The cruellest legacy of my acne is the profound conviction that I am different to others' (cited in Lansdown et al. 1997: 61).

The feeling of difference can be regularly reinforced by the behaviour of others. Marc Crank described this experience with great eloquence:

> The disfigured person often cannot hide or disguise their 'difference' and must wear it like a badge. All too frequently complete strangers regard the fact that one looks different as a sign that they can walk up to you and demand intimate details about your disfigurement. It seems that they believe they have a right to ask personal questions whether they know you or not.
>
> (Lansdown et al. 1997: 28)

He recalls a particularly galling experience when visiting the Tower of London, when strangers started talking about him within his earshot: 'They were so intrigued that they rounded up as many of their friends, relatives and anyone else that was interested to join their group and continue staring, pointing and discussing me'. MacGregor (1974) described these behaviours as visual or verbal 'assaults'. People with visible differences may feel deprived of the ability to manage the information relating to the self that others derive from physical appearance, and feel unable to control the initial assumptions and misconceptions other people make about the sort of person they are.

In addition to unwanted invasions of privacy, research has established that there are other tangible differences in the behaviour of others when encountering someone with a visible difference (see Newell (2000b) and Bull and Rumsey (1988) for more comprehensive reviews of these studies). Rumsey et al. (1982) established that strangers leave a greater physical distance between themselves and a stranger with a facial disfigurement than between themselves and the same person without a disfigurement. In a study of seat occupancy on underground trains, Houston and Bull (1994) demonstrated that the seat next to a person with a facial birthmark was left empty significantly more often than when the same person appeared without a disfigurement. When approached by a 'market researcher' with a facial disfigurement, fewer people agreed to answer questions than when the same person approached passers-by without a disfigurement (Rumsey et al. 1986). However, the results of studies of altruism were intriguing, as in studies which did not involve face-to-face contact (for example, posting a 'lost' application form complete with passport photo) respondents were equally helpful whether or not the person needing help was visibly different. When face-to-face interaction was required, fewer people agreed to initiate an encounter with a person with a facial birthmark, but once engaged, they were subsequently more helpful than participants interacting with the same person without a facial difference (Rumsey et al. 1986).

Explanations for the behaviour of others have been many and various, and have included the notion that beliefs in a 'just world' cause people to imagine that the person with a visible difference must have deserved their 'fate', and can therefore be derogated or avoided (Novak and Lerner 1968). Evolutionary perspectives have also proposed an innate aversion to anything other than perfect. Gilbert (1997) has argued that as with other vertebrates, our reactions towards others are guided by our perceptions of their relative ranking in society, that social attractiveness counts highly in this process and people will seek to form alliances with those perceived as socially attractive and to avoid those perceived as unattractive. Alternatively, a lack of knowledge may result in the desire to avoid anything that might be contagious (Bernstein 1976), or avoidance due to uncertainty about how to behave (Langer et al. 1976; see also Bull and Rumsey 1988 for a more detailed review). These explanations are clearly simplistic, and the weight both of research evidence and personal accounts suggests that the responses of others are affected by a combination of factors, including initial stereotyping during the impression formation stage of an encounter, an uncertainty of how to behave due to a lack of previous experience, and the tendency to avoid an encounter to minimize potential embarrassment to oneself, or the person with a difference.

### The behaviour of people with visible differences

Social encounters may also be thrown off-kilter by the physical limitations to non-verbal expression caused by a facial difference or by other aspects of the behaviour of the person with the visible difference. An inability to use facial musculature in the usual ways (for example as the result of a facial palsy, or in the case of Moebious syndrome which inhibits the facial expression of emotion) will lead to unconventional facial expressions and difficulties for others in 'reading' the faces of people with visible differences (MacGregor 1989). This is likely to result in hesitancy and awkwardness for other parties in the interaction. Discomfort on either side may contribute to an unsatisfactory or abbreviated interchange.

The avoidant or stilted reactions of others may result in negative spirals of aversive emotional responses, maladaptive thought processes (including social anxiety and fear of negative social evaluation by others), unfavourable self-perceptions (for example, lowered self-esteem or unfavourable body image) and behaviour patterns (for example, excessive use of social avoidance and heavy reliance on concealment of the disfigurement) for the affected person. Negative experiences in social situations can lead to an understandable preoccupation with the effect a disfigurement has on others and the assumption that negative reactions will result in most social situations. MacGregor (1979) talked of those affected being acutely aware of the responses of others, and expending excessive amounts of energy attending to these reactions. The result may be a less than optimal interaction style, which can manifest in outright social avoidance, shyness, awkwardness and embarrass-ment, defensiveness or hostility towards others. Kathy Wheatley said that she 'came across as overconfident and brash. It's overcompensation. If you are pretty you forget how much you use that as a form of communication. Now I have to rely on my personality' (cited in Lansdown et al. 1997: 183).

Adachi et al. (2003) videoed interactions and examined the head and hand movements and frequency of smiling in adult women with or without a cleft lip and palate. They found that cleft-affected participants displayed significantly fewer head nods, and a lower smile frequency than the control group. They also concluded that the head and hand movements and smiles occurred with less synchrony than the non-cleft participants.

A laboratory-based study published by Rumsey and her colleagues in 1986 lent credence to the potential power of the behaviour of the affected person to influence the process and outcome of interactions with others. For the purposes of experimental control, the person studied had an artificially applied 'facial birthmark' and was trained to interact with par-ticipants using a high or low level of social skill. Posing as a trainee clinical psychologist practising interviewing techniques, interactions with a series of participants were videoed and analysed. The verbal and non-verbal com-munication displayed by participants in the 'disfigured/high skill' condition was the most positive and the impressions formed by the participants of the interviewer in this condition were the most favourable. The behaviour and ratings of participants were least favourable in the disfigured/low skill condition, with the results for the non-disfigured/high skill ranking second, and non-disfigured/low skill, third. The results offered a promising avenue in the search for effective methods of promoting more positive experiences of social interactions.

*Visible difference and personal relationships*

In addition to difficulties in initial interactions with strangers, some people with disfigurements report a negative impact of their appearance on longer-term relationships. Kent (1999) has discussed problems which may result from a deprivation of touch in those with skin conditions, and has specu-lated about links made to a subsequent lowering of self-esteem. Some studies have reported concealment of a disfigurement from close friends and even partners; for example, Lanigan and Cotterill (1989) reported that 9 per cent of their female sample concealed their birthmarks even from partners. When a difference is acquired in the context of an established relationship, the problems often relate to the person with the disfigurement. Gamba et al. (1992) reported a worsened sexual relationship with partners after surgical treatment for head and neck cancer in 74 per cent of patients. Porter et al. (1990) explored the sexual relationships of people with vitiligo. Half the respondents who reported a decrease in sexual activity said this was due to their own anxiety and discomfort rather than the reactions of partners.

Ramsey and O'Reagan (1988) found that 50 per cent of their sample of people with psoriasis reported similar effects.

There have been reports that people affected by a cleft lip and palate may marry at a later age than their non-cleft peers, and that they may experience less marital satisfaction than controls (Peter and Chinsky 1974). There has been speculation that negative self-evaluations may lead some people with visible differences to settle for the wrong partner, as they fear their alternatives may be limited. John Storry, who was born with a significant jaw malformation movingly wrote:

> I am intelligent and sensitive but I have to accept that I cannot have a deep, satisfying and intimate relationship . . . I cannot be loved and I cannot love . . . I am told that personality is more important than surface appearance. The statement is correct but it overlooks one critical factor. I think it is impossible to develop an attractive personality with a damaged face.
>
> (cited in Lansdown et al. 1997: 33)

Although research has in the main focused on the difficulties associated with establishing and maintaining satisfying friendships and relationships, these experiences are by no means universal within the population of people with visible differences. The factors which appear to increase or reduce the risk of problematic social experiences are explored in Chapter 5.

*Older adults*

Research examining the impact of disfigurements on older adults is very limited. Increasing life expectancy and improvements in health care mean that ever-larger numbers of older people are living with visible differences, or alterations to appearance caused by surgical or medical treatments. In the absence of research evidence, increasing age is assumed by many to confer protection against concerns about appearance. However, in an unpublished thesis, Spicer (2002) reported data that showed the picture to be more complex than this. Seventy adult attendees at a dermatology clinic aged 65 or over completed standardized measures and a semi-structured interview. In comparison to scores for young and middle-aged adults attending a similar clinic, mean levels of anxiety, social anxiety and social avoidance were lower for the older group; however, there was marked variation within the sample and over one-third reported that they were experiencing high levels of appearance-related distress and concern. Feelings of embarrassment and self-consciousness and reports of avoidance of social activities and negative effects on relationships were common among this group. Most of the older participants felt that 'appearances' were still important; however, they also reported that the focus of their concern had shifted from a desire to look 'attractive', to one of 'propriety' – the wish to appear clean, tidy and smart. Many felt that their appearance concerns were not fully appreciated by clinicians. When planning improvements to care provision (: 7), the needs of older adults should not be overlooked.

### Disfigurement as an underlying stressor across the lifespan

Lansdown et al. (1997) described disfigurement and its treatment as an underlying stressor in the daily lives of those affected, and Middleton (personal communication) has further developed this idea and applied it to the whole lifespan. A visible difference can be conceptualized as a continuous stressor, one which makes continuous calls on energy reserves and coping resources. The percentage of time it occupies can vary from a relatively small amount, when other aspects of life are going well, to all-consuming proportions, for example following its initial onset, or at times of surgical intervention. When other life stresses and strains occur (whether typical of a particular life stage, or resulting from a significant event such as a relationship break-up), the disfigurement may increase in salience, and in some cases, may become the focus or 'hook' for other difficulties. Clinical experience suggests that times of transition can be particularly hard for those with a visible difference throughout the lifespan, particularly transitions which result in changing social groups (for example, moving house, changing schools; leaving school/home; starting at college, university or a new job; changing jobs, beginning and ending relationships and so on). These transitions provide a useful focus for effective support and intervention (see Chapters 6 and 7).

### Condition-specific effects

Although the commonalities in the experiences of people with a broad range of visible differences are striking, there are also some specific effects which occur as the result of particular conditions. As the causes of disfigurement are many and various, comprehensive coverage of all these condition-specific effects is beyond the scope of this review. Accordingly, we have chosen examples which give a flavour of the enormous range of conditions to which appearance research is relevant – and those areas in which there is sufficient research to feel reasonably confident of the conclusions. The bulk of research relating to congenital conditions has concerned cleft lip/palate. As this research has been well represented in the preceding sections on lifespan issues, it is not duplicated here.

### Cancer

In addition to the fear of a potentially life-threatening condition, many people with cancer are severely distressed by disruption and changes to their appearance as a result of disease and its treatment.

Some cancer-related changes to appearance are temporary (for example, hair loss) or amenable to change (such as with reconstructive surgery after mastectomy), while others are permanent (amputation) and may impact on functioning in addition to appearance (White 2002). Changes to appearance can act as vivid, constant reminders of the disease and its treatment and the fear that the cancer might return (White 2002). Generally, the incidence of body image problems among patients with cancer is not well documented and the personal impact of changes to appearance may well be underestimated, possibly because patients fear that it would be inappropriate to report such concerns when their focus should be upon survival and efforts to conquer the disease (Hopwood and Maguire 1988).

Much of the available research has focused upon body image and appearance among patients with head and neck cancer, breast cancer or stoma, with other diagnoses receiving relatively little attention. Since cancer patients are a diverse and heterogenous group (Zabora et al. 2001), more research is needed to consider the specific appearance-related concerns of different diagnostic, prognostic and treatment groups. To date, the appearance-related impact of non-malignant conditions has been largely overlooked in the research literature but may be a major concern for those affected, as patients may still undergo treatment that could result in scarring akin to that experienced by those with a confirmed malignancy. The NHS breast screening programme in the UK has led to an increase in the number of women diagnosed as having ductal carcinoma in situ (DCIS), a pre-invasive condition that may or may not evolve into breast cancer at a later stage. Women diagnosed with DCIS essentially have two choices: they can 'wait and see' whether they develop full-blown breast cancer or they can choose to have the area of DCIS surgically removed through mastectomy or lumpectomy (with or without radiotherapy and/or reconstructive surgery). Thus, although women are reassured that they do not yet have a malignancy, they are offered treatment that is synonymous with breast cancer and which can have a major impact upon body image and appearance. While the limited available research in this area has focused on satisfaction with information, support and care provided (Bluman et al. 2001; Brown et al. 2000; De Morgan et al. 2002), our research (Harcourt and Griffiths 2003) has focused on the threat and dilemma that this presents, including the impact on appearance:

> I've had friends with cancer and they've all had lumpectomies . . .
> I never in a million years thought I'd have to have a mastectomy, so
> my reaction wasn't really to the diagnosis, my reaction was to the
> mastectomy.

The most common forms of treatment for cancer (surgery, chemotherapy, radiotherapy and drug/hormone therapy) all have the potential to impact upon appearance:

*Surgery*

Many patients undergo a series of surgical procedures in order to diagnose and remove a malignant tumour and, subsequently, reconstructive surgery in attempts to restore their pre-surgical appearance and/or functioning (see Chapter 6). Radical surgery will result in scarring and in addition can also cause loss of function, lymphoedema (swelling) and the need to rely on prostheses or appliances (for example, stoma). It is often presumed that more extensive surgery will have a greater psychological impact than less invasive or mutilating surgery. For example, a body of literature has found that women with breast cancer who undergo lumpectomy (surgical removal of the tumour and surrounding tissue) report more favourable post-surgical body image and greater satisfaction with their bodies than do women who undergo mastectomy (complete removal of the breast tissue) (see King et al. 2000; Moyer 1997). However, a lumpectomy still results in scarring and can have an obvious impact on appearance and body image (Hall and Fallowfield 1989) and patients who elect lumpectomy over mastectomy in the belief that less radical surgery will not change the appearance of their breasts may be disappointed (Fallowfield and Clarke 1991).

*Chemotherapy*

Rapid alopecia (hair loss) is often a particularly traumatic experience and is, for many, the most feared side effect of chemotherapy (Batchelor 2001). Rosman (2004) reported a qualitative study of patients' experiences of chemo-induced hair loss, illustrating how changes in appearance had increased participants' sense of identity as cancer patients and their concern that their illness was now public knowledge. Hair loss was seen as a stigmatizing event, but for many it was 'the price to be paid for being cured' (p. 336). Using wigs in order to disguise and camouflage this change may not be a simple solution, since some patients report that wigs feel unnatural, serve to emphasize feelings of difference (Williams et al. 1999) and raise issues as to when to disclose the hair loss (Rosman 2004). The negative impact of chemotherapy may ameliorate as hair starts to regrow (Pendley et al. 1997) but patients may have to make further adjustment to an altered appearance if the new growth is a different texture and colour.

Chemotherapy can also result in significant weight changes that can prove particularly difficult to hide or disguise and feelings of nausea and vomiting that might be perceived as an indication of a recurrence or another cancer (Price 1992). In addition, patients may find the means by which chemotherapy is administered (for example, Hickman lines and frequent injections) both intrusive and threatening to body integrity.

*Radiotherapy*

The extreme fatigue commonly associated with radiotherapy treatment may conflict with daily functioning, with consequences for body image. These side effects may also be interpreted as symptoms of the ongoing presence of cancer. In addition, some patients suffer skin reactions to radiotherapy that can take considerable time to heal and may result in permanent scarring.

*Hormonal therapy*

Steroids and hormonal therapy designed to stem the growth of a malignant tumour can have a distressing impact on appearance. For example, the side effects of drugs used as standard treatment for breast cancer may involve menopausal-like symptoms including weight gain and hot flushes. Patients with prostate cancer treated by hormonal therapy have reported how treatment-induced changes in their appearance create a physical and emotional distance between them and their spouses (Navon and Morag 2003).

In summary, all forms of cancer treatment have the potential to detrimentally affect aspects of body appearance, sensation and function. These processes may be compounded for those patients who undergo a combination of treatments. The precise impact for any individual is difficult to predict. While many patients consider an altered appearance to be a relatively small price to pay for treatment of a life-threatening condition, for others this is a particularly traumatic aspect of their disease. Researchers and clinicians working in this area have been criticized for failing to consider the importance of the personal value attached to the part of the body affected by the cancer (White 2002; see also Chapter 2). There is much more to be learned about the impact of treatment-related changes to body image and how these might be ameliorated (see Chapters 6 and 7).

### Burns (with contributions from Claire Phillips)

Although a few burn injuries are premeditated (for example as a variant of self-harm), the vast majority happen suddenly and unexpectedly. Approximately 175,000 people in the UK present at an Accident & Emergency department with burn injuries each year and 13,000 of those are admitted to hospital (National Burn Care Review Committee Report 2001). Compared to other forms of traumatic injury, burns have a greater propensity to cause widespread damage, dysfunction and disfigurement and the sudden and rapid changes to appearance resulting from burn injury present a number of unique challenges. In addition, the cause of the accident resulting in the burn may be attributable to the actions, or non-actions of the patient, family member or other people present at the event. The emotions and stress associated with the circumstances surrounding the injury may be hard to resolve.

A person with a burn injury will typically go through a series of treatment stages following the accident. The first task after the emergency management of the event is to close the open wounds using skin grafts or by promoting the regeneration of skin. This period is typified by the need to control infection and pain and by repeated stressful dressing changes. Wounds typically look raw and unpleasant and patients and parents may experience disbelief that even a seemingly small accident (such as spilling a cup of tea) could cause such severe and widespread damage. Patients and families have to accept that although the burns or scalds look severe in the early post-burn phase, they will improve. Patients may initially be discouraged from looking at facial burns until the swelling has reduced and the fierceness of the burn has calmed. In this phase, patients may be watching for clues to the extent of their injuries from the reactions of visiting relatives and friends: 'I did kind of look for things once I found out that I'd lost my hair and stuff like that. I kind of wanted to gauge people's reactions' (female, 22 years).

A burn-injured person may be referred to a Scar Management Team to try and minimize the undesirable aspects of burn scars (their raised appearance or the restriction of movement due to scarring). This may involve wearing specially tailored, tight-fitting pressure garments designed to prevent the scar from overgrowing and becoming lumpy in appearance. Ironically, while pressure garments are designed to help minimize the appearance of the scar tissue, this ongoing treatment can itself become a source of curiosity for the general public. Pressure garments worn over facial burns can resemble masks, and can provoke particularly noticeable reactions from others. Levels of adherence to the prescribed use of pressure garments may be compromised by a dislike of their appearance.

After what may be a lengthy period of hospitalization, concerns about the appearance of the burn may come to the fore as patients return home and face the reactions of others to their altered appearance:

> I did get fed up of answering the same thing and explaining. You feel that when you meet somebody, you've got to tell them all about your accident, because at the end they're going to ask a question and you've got to talk about the accident.
>
> (male, 48 years)

> And after the accident, she wouldn't come near me, which hurt. She [granddaughter] was scared stiff, seeing me as I was like.
>
> (male, 53 years)

There may be concerns the burns may be misinterpreted as contagious:

> I don't want people being put off going in the swimming pool simply because (pause) I've jumped in the water and they're thinking, yuk,

what might I catch off him, sort of thing. You know, it's easy for other people to misunderstand.

(male, 39 years)

The burned person or the parent of a burned child might try to hide their burns with clothing in order to fend off questions and looks or stares. Additionally, the burn site should be protected from sunlight as the new skin is extremely fragile and sensitive to damaging UV rays. A person can therefore feel conspicuous by their seasonally incongruent clothing such as long trousers or sleeves or by generous amounts of sunblock.

The appearance of the burn injury changes gradually for the first 18 months to two years as scars mature and become stable. Colour fades and scars become less rigid and obvious. However, during this maturation period the eventual outcome is uncertain and anxiety about the current and future appearance of the scars is common. During the process of change, the affected person may be buoyed up by the hope that the scars will look better by the end of treatment. Expectations of the eventual outcome may be unrealistic and adaptation to the altered appearance may be inadvertently delayed. In addition, scars are likely to be a permanent reminder of the trauma associated with injury and treatment: 'The odd time I'll look at him, he'll be in the bath or whatever, and I think, you know, it's just like a constant reminder sometimes and you see him, and you think I wish he could have smooth skin' (Mother of Patient, male, 2 years).

In Claire Phillips' sample of 66 burn-injured adults, levels of social functioning explained 76 per cent of the variance in psychological functioning post-burn ($\beta$ = +0.6, p<0.01) and self-ratings of attractiveness were the second strongest predictor for psychological functioning ($\beta$ = +0.4, p<0.01). Levels of appearance anxiety (measured by the Derriford Appearance Scale) were greater in a sample of burned adults compared to a general population sample (z = 2.05, p = 0.02). While early return to work has been demonstrated to be an indicator of good adjustment (Questad et al. 1988) those affected may feel that their altered appearance will affect their job situation through reducing their desire to do public-facing jobs, undermining their chances of promotion or causing them to stay in a familiar job where they are already known:

I think that it would make it harder for me to be confident in interviews and to come across that way . . . erm . . . because I'm quite self-conscious about the way I look. And so I think that would hinder me, but also I think that . . . erm . . . people might look at me and kind of judge me on the way I look and not be as happy to give me a job or kind of just because of that . . . I wouldn't be as ready to change firms just because I'd be more secure with the people that I kind of know and understand what's happened to me.

(female, 22 years)

Despite these issues, research indicates that many return to their former roles and adjust with varying levels of success to their previous life (Blakeney et al. 1988; Meyers-Paal et al. 2000). Adjustment to burns is a multifaceted and complex process occurring over time and involving a combination of social factors, characteristics intrinsic to the individual (such as personality, resilience, outlook and optimism), individual features of the burn (such as location and visibility and the circumstances under which it was acquired), the affected person's perception of the severity and noticeability of the burn to others (Kleve and Robinson 1999), and the level or extent of surgical intervention required (see Chapter 5).

*Skin conditions*

The skin is the largest organ of the body. Its condition reflects our general health status and can indicate a range of difficulties including emotional stress, allergic reactions, lack of sleep, poor diet or eating habits. Papadopoulos et al. describe it as 'a door to physical and psychological problems and processes' (1999b: 108). It is a visible gauge by which we can judge other people and be judged ourselves. Disfiguring skin conditions may be congenital or acquired and, contrary to popular stereotypes are not the sole preserve of adolescents. The prevalence of disorders increases with age and it has been reported that 10 per cent of people aged over 70 suffer from 10 to 15 skin complaints simultaneously (Kligman 1989).

Skin conditions can be progressive (as in vitiligo) or fluctuating. The lack of predictability about the course of most dermatological conditions is problematic for many, as this means that those affected must be prepared for possible deterioration and flare ups of the condition at any time. Yet, since the majority of skin conditions are unlikely to be life threatening (Papadopoulos et al. 1999) they are often seen by health care professionals as a predominantly cosmetic problem. As such their psychosocial impact may not be fully appreciated and is often trivialized. Koo (1995) has suggested that the psychosocial effects of acne are the most distressing aspects of the disease for the majority of patients and it seems reasonable to suggest that this applies equally to many other skin conditions.

While some psychosocial issues (for example, social anxiety and social avoidance) are pertinent across the range of dermatological conditions, it is also important that additional condition-specific issues (for example, the fragility of the skin and problems of touch in the skin blistering condition, epidermolysis bullosa (EB)) are not overlooked. Skin conditions which involve blistering, flaking or scaly skin, such as eczema and psoriasis, may mean that it is difficult for those affected to use make up to conceal their condition. A greater reliance is put on the use of clothing, yet this may bring its own problems (for example, covering arms and legs in summer; Porter et al. 1986; see also Chapter 6 about camouflage services).

The possible links between stress and the progression of skin conditions has been the subject of much recent interest. Papadopoulos et al. (1998) conducted a retrospective, cross-sectional study to examine the impact of life events on the onset of vitiligo in adults. The number of stressful life events occurring over the previous year were compared with a control group consisting of other appearance-altering conditions (dystropic epidermolysis bullosa and naevi), chosen because they are not considered to be associated with stress. Those with vitiligo had experienced a significantly higher proportion of life events than the matched controls. This led the authors to conclude that people are born with a genetic predisposition for the condition which may be precipitated by the trauma of a stressful life event. While this interpretation assumes that all those who experienced a particular life event found it stressful and fails to consider individual appraisals of stress and coping, it offers support for the inclusion of stress management in any comprehensive care provision (see Chapter 7).

### Rheumatoid arthritis

Rheumatoid arthritis (RA) is characterized by pain, loss of functional ability, uncertainty about progression and altered appearance including swelled joints. However, relatively little attention has been paid to issues relating to body image and appearance issues in those affected by this chronic condition. Exceptionally, Rumsey et al.'s (2002) study explored the appearance concerns of 57 outpatients with rheumatic conditions. They reported that levels of anxiety and depression were higher than for many other groups of patients with visible conditions, including burns, head and neck cancer and eye conditions. Those reporting higher levels of distress talked of embarrassment about the appearance of their joints, and with lesions and discoloration of the skin. They felt their condition was very noticeable to others, resulting in acute self-consciousness. Seventy-two per cent reported avoiding various activities, including swimming, trying on clothes in communal changing rooms, and the curtailing of social activities.

Vamos (1990) investigated the importance of body image concerns relating to the appearance of the hand among 80 female outpatients with RA. Participants commented that the appearance of their hands had evoked responses from others, for example pitying glances similar to the negative experiences reported by people with a facial difference. Participants recalled feelings of shame or anger as a result. Negative feelings about the appearance of arthritic hands were significant predictors of desire for surgery independently of age, duration of condition, grip strength and objectively rated hand appearance. In contrast to the emphasis of research into facial differences, there has been relatively little attention paid to conditions in which hands are affected (see Rumsey 2003b). Yet, like the face, hands are very visible in social interaction, and their appearance can be difficult to cover unobtrusively.

Ben-Tovim and Walker (1995) investigated body-related attitudes of women with long-standing acquired or congenital disorders affecting body appearance or functioning. Their study included women with RA (who were classified as 'disfigured and disabled'); skin conditions (deemed 'disfigured but not disabled'); a group with visible blood vessel deformities including port wine stains and a group with diabetes. All participants were female because the Body Attitudes Questionnaire (BAQ) used in this study was developed for use with women. Comparisons were made with participants from a large random community sample of South Australian women matched on age, weight and height, none of whom had manifest disabling or disfiguring disorders of comparable severity to those in the clinical groups. All condition groups felt less attractive to the other sex than matched controls but this difference was only significant among the diabetes group. Among those with RA, younger age of onset was significantly correlated with more intense disparagement of the body and concerns about weight and shape. The primary determinant of body attitudes was age of onset rather than duration of illness, with those whose condition emerged during early adolescence reporting more intense negative body appraisal. Participants who were diagnosed as having JRA (juvenile onset rheumatoid arthritis) felt subjectively fatter than their same weight community counterparts and had a widespread incidence of negative appraisals of their own bodies. The authors suggested that appropriate psychological interventions including support for appearance concerns might be beneficial for individuals with RA, especially those diagnosed in adolescence.

### Tattooing

Permanent skin markings have been used as a way of customizing the body for centuries, although the term was first used in the eighteenth century (MacLachlan 2004). Having previously been associated with rebelliousness and possibly indicative of group membership and socioeconomic status, tattoos are now seen by increasing numbers as acceptable (MacLachlan 2004). The numbers of tattooing parlours in the UK have increased from 100 twenty years ago to 1500 in 2004 – even Barbie now sports a tattoo on her abdomen. Motivations for tattooing are complex and include a desire for body modification, self-expression and creativity, yet acquiring a tattoo carries with it health risks in terms of mild blood poisoning, possible infections and the transmission of diseases which may be potentially lethal (for example in relation to HIV or Hepatitis C) (Armstrong and Murphy 1997). Subsequently, a sizeable proportion of people regret their decision to have a permanent tattoo and express a strong desire for their removal. Removal of a tattoo, by way of laser, dermabrasion or cutting, can be prolonged, painful and expensive. It will not necessarily eradicate all evidence of the tattoo and an individual is likely to be trading the tattoo for an area of scarring.

High levels of appearance-related distress and regret were found in Rumsey et al.'s (2004) sample of 25 people attending a privately funded tattoo removal clinic. Participants reported strikingly high levels of general anxiety, social avoidance and social anxiety that were significantly greater than those found in patients affected by burns, head and neck cancer and skin conditions. Feelings of self-consciousness and embarrassment were common, and the majority felt that their tattoos resulted in negative stereotyping by others.

## Conclusion

In summary, a visible disfigurement presents a variety of significant challenges. Although visible differences are caused by an enormous range of conditions, there are more similarities than differences in the experiences of those affected, regardless of the aetiology. The commonality in the experiences of all people with appearance concerns – whether or not these are the result of an objective disfigurement – is also striking, with the most frequently reported issues relating to negative self-perceptions and difficulties in social interactions. Although researchers exploring the concerns of the general population and those working in the field of disfigurement have treated these as separate areas in the past, there are strong arguments for considering appearance concerns across the broad population spectrum in future.

The literature concerning the effects of visible differences paints a picture of those affected being more at risk for body image concerns, low self-esteem and social interaction problems; however, not all are equally affected. Estimates of the proportion who experience significant psychological disturbance vary according to the participant population (those actively seeking treatment, or samples drawn from community settings), the sample size (often very small) and the measures used (see Chapter 2; Newell 2000a). However, most studies agree that between 30 and 50 per cent of those attending for hospital treatment experience significant levels of appearance-related distress. Studies have also shown, however, that others cope effectively and relegate their difference to a minor role, with some developing the belief that they can use their difference to good advantage (Partridge 1990; Rumsey 2002a). In a qualitative study, 46 per cent of a sample of limb amputees believed that something good had happened as the result of their amputation (Gallager and MacLachlan 2000). Themes included the belief that the experience had changed respondents' attitudes to life, increased their confidence, patience and levels of contentment, and had promoted the development of more effective coping abilities. Several mentioned that the experience had been 'character building'. In the midst of all the negative press associated with psoriasis, Ginsberg and Link (1989) offered evidence of a positive attitude in some of those affected. In contrast to others with the same condition, these people disagreed with the notion that they were rejected by others in their social circle because of their skin condition, and were characterized by a pervading sense of optimism concerning many aspects of their lives.

Although to ease our fevered research brains it is tempting to dichotomize those affected by disfigurement as predominantly 'positive' or 'negative' copers, clearly a complex interplay of experiences characterizes the daily experiences of many. Andrews (1998) has argued that people can hold both positive self-attitudes and negative ones, and that self-esteem can fluctuate over time and situations. The extent to which people fluctuate between relative adjustment and distress remains to be explored, yet although a detailed understanding of these processes may be some years away, researchers have begun to detail the evidence for factors which seem to exacerbate distress or buffer people against appearance-related concerns. These are explored more fully in Chapter 5.

## Chapter summary

♦ Drawing boundaries around what does and does not constitute a disfigurement is far from straightforward;
♦ Visible differences can result from a large variety of causes, including congenital and acquired abnormalities, trauma, disease and the aftermath of surgery;
♦ The most common problems experienced by people with visible differences relate to negative self-perceptions, fear of negative evaluations by others and difficulties with social interactions;
♦ Between 30 and 50 per cent of people attending hospitals for the treatment of disfiguring conditions experience significant psychological problems in relation to their appearance;
♦ Problems can be affected by developmental stage and by some condition-specific effects, but the similarities in the problems experienced by people with different sorts of disfigurements are greater than the differences.

## Discussion points

♦ How would you define disfigurement?
♦ If you had a very noticeable facial difference, how would you handle an encounter with a stranger?
♦ What are the similarities and differences in the nature and impact of appearance concerns of people with and without objective disfigurements?

**Further reading**

Endriga, M.C. and Kapp-Simon, K.A. (1999) Psychological issues in craniofacial care: state of the art. *The Cleft Palate-Craniofacial Journal*, 36: 3–9.
Lansdown, R., Rumsey, N., Bradbury, E., Carr, T. and Partridge, J. (1997) *Visibly Different: Coping with Disfigurement*. Oxford: Butterworth-Heinemann.
Newell, R. (2000a) *Body Image and Disfigurement Care*. London: Routledge.
Rumsey, N. and Harcourt, D. (2004) Body image and disfigurement: issues and interventions. *Body Image*, 1. 83–97.

# Psychological predictors of vulnerability and resilience

Research in the area of appearance concerns, whether experienced by people with visible differences or by the broader public, has in the main focused on negative experiences, highlighting the debilitating nature of the problems experienced. However, it has become increasingly clear that this is only part of the story; for example, 70 per cent of respondents to a survey of members of the Cleft Lip and Palate Association in the UK reported positive consequences of having a cleft lip and/or palate (Cochrane and Slade 1999). Strauss (2001) has posed the question of why, in spite of the numerous challenges and problems demonstrated in the literature, many people with craniofacial conditions become productive, contributing, happy, satisfied individuals. Clearly, although a disfigurement has the potential to dominate the life of an affected person, a substantial proportion cope well. In recent years, the impetus towards considering positive experiences has been growing. The momentum has gathered from several sources, notably from some articulate advocates of people with disfigurements who feel that an exclusive focus on the problems and difficulties contributes to a view of disfigurement which is unhelpful, as it is both pathologizing and negative. In addition, appearance researchers in the UK and the USA have been intrigued by the quest to unravel the tangle of factors contributing to adjustment for some time.

## An alternative to the pathologizing approach

Crucial to explaining individual differences in adjustment is the need to identify protective factors that act as buffers to excessive or debilitating appearance concerns, and those predisposing factors that make individuals especially vulnerable to social and cultural pressures regarding appearance. Without understanding the intricacies of adjustment, we can offer only blunt aids to more positive coping and better health care provision. Eiserman (2001) believes that we also have an ethical obligation to consider the positive aspects of life with disfigurement. He argues that decisions about policy and care should not be made just on the basis of those with problems, but on a balanced depiction of life with a visible difference. One particularly interesting related debate surrounds the issue of the measures used in research (see Chapter 2). The majority of current scales can be construed as negative, focusing on psychological morbidity and dysfunction. Many of the researchers within the CAR feel uneasy about using these scales, as their hunch is that if participants weren't feeling depressed before they answered the questions, the likelihood is that they would by the time they had finished! A research focus which embraces positive as well as negative experiences brings with it the need to develop new, more balanced measures.

In view of the extensive commonalities between the experience of people with and without disfigurements (see Chapters 3 and 4), where appropriate, the factors affecting resilience and distress for both populations will be considered together in this chapter. An appealing by-product of this approach is the ability to locate the concerns of those people with visible differences in the context of 'normative' levels of discontent and appearance concern in the mainstream population, rather than classifying people with visible differences as a separate 'abnormal' group.

## Resilience

In attempts to explain the processes which appear to buffer a person against the stresses and strains of living with a visible difference, the attention of several appearance researchers has focused on the attribute of 'resilience'. Cooper (2000) defined resilience in the context of disfigurement as 'the ability to develop the self confidence to withstand the social and psycho-logical pressures', or alternatively, 'the ability to take the hard knocks, weather the storm and continue to value oneself whatever happens'. Bradbury (personal communication) has developed the appealing analogy of resilience as a kind of force field around a person – an impervious layer which causes negative reactions from others and the omnipresent media messages extolling the benefits of beauty to rebound harmlessly.

The components of resilience have been described in various ways, although common general themes emerge. Mouradian (2001) outlined the 'essential' components of resilience as being positive self-beliefs, effective social skills and social support, as in her view, these factors distinguish those who cope well with craniofacial anomalies from those who experience more debilitating problems. In a series of 18 telephone interviews involving people with facial paralysis, Meyerson (2001) identified family support, faith, humour, sense of self, special skills, determination and networking as influencing resilience. In an unpublished qualitative interview study with eight participants, Wright (2002) identified three major themes characterizing positive coping: a 'resilient personality' (including confidence, a high level of sociability, good sense of humour and a predisposition to relish a challenge); high-quality social support from family and friends, which emphasized normality rather than difference; and lastly, effective social skills. She found no notable differences in the themes derived from people with congenital or acquired disfigurements.

In relation to body image, Thompson et al.'s (2002) authoritative review of the variables that may account for individual differences includes coverage of a huge array of societal and social factors, interpersonal influences including the influence of peers, parents and strangers together with behavioural and cognitive self processes.

Using data derived from a general population sample, Carr (2004) proposed four contributory aspects of the self-system which were associated with low levels of appearance concern, namely strong self-esteem, self-efficacy, 'functional' coping strategies (which Carr proposed as including an optimistic attributional style, effective social support, positive use of meditation and relaxation, exercise, and the cognitive strategies of problem solving, reframing and distraction), 'adaptive defences', and a future-oriented perspective on life. Carr (2004) also refers to trait theory and argues that this research has led to the identification of a highly resilient personality profile characterized by positive adjustment on all the NEO5 factors: extraversion (good social adjustment and success in interpersonal relationships); high levels of emotional stability (good mental and physical health); openness to experience (associated with creativity and absorption); agreeableness (associated with altruism and good interpersonal relationships); and conscientiousness (predictive of good academic and occupational performance). Carr speculates that there are neurobiological correlates associated with this personality type, and also outlines the links to subjective wellbeing.

Work in this area is still in its infancy – and may feel bewildering to the uninitiated – for example, among the issues yet to be resolved is whether resilience should be seen as a personality trait or as a coping strategy or resource. Is it inherited? Which aspects can be taught or acquired? More investment is needed in this promising area. The payoffs of increasing understanding are billed as likely to be considerable, as many believe that at least some of the relevant skills can be learned and/or further developed. The UK based charity Changing Faces for example, is eager for research to inform its work. A key aim of the charity is to equip people who seek their help with three types of resilience:

♦ behavioural resilience (the capacity to interact successfully with others, and to manage their reactions to a visible difference);
♦ cognitive resilience (the capacity to use self-talk in a supportive and

positive way, constantly challenging one's own assumptions that looking different means a second class existence);
♦ emotional resilience (the capacity to feel good about oneself and one's ability to cope successfully with difficulties).

However, before we all leap on to the 'resilience' bandwagon, another side of the coin should be considered. Is there a potential danger of focusing too much on the universal desirability of a particular kind of resilience? This approach might develop into a form of value judgement preached by the converted (and well adjusted), which pressurizes people to cope in a particular way, and may result in guilt if this particular type of positive adjustment is not achieved.

## Factors exacerbating or ameliorating distress

With these provisos in mind, work continues to identify those factors which exacerbate or ameliorate distress and promote positive coping. In the next section, these have been grouped broadly into:

♦ physical and treatment-related factors (including the aetiology, extent, type and severity of the visible difference, and the treatment history);
♦ demographic and sociocultural factors (including age and developmental stage, gender, race, social class and cultural milieu, together with the influence of parents, peers and the media); and
♦ psychological factors and processes (including self-esteem and self-image, the weight given to the perceived opinions of others, cognitive processes, and perceived levels of social support).

### The aetiology and physical characteristics of a visible difference

Contrary to the expectations of the lay public and many health care providers, the bulk of research, clinical experience and personal accounts demonstrate that the extent, type and severity of a disfigurement consistently fail to predict adjustment (Rumsey and Harcourt 2004). A person's individual subjective perception of how noticeable his or her difference is to others is a better predictor of psychological and body image disturbance than the assessment of a dispassionate observer or clinician (Harris 1997).

There has been a continual thread of debate in the literature concerning the role played in body image distress and psychosocial adjustment by the aetiology of the visible difference, with some writers particularly keen to generalize about the impact of effects caused by disfigurements present from birth, and those acquired later in life. Newell (2000a), who has provided a useful review and methodological critique of relevant studies, avoided this simplistic distinction. He maintained that there is a consistent finding of less disturbance among people disfigured from birth or from accidental injury compared with those affected by skin conditions, or with disfiguration resulting from surgery. However, the numbers of relevant studies are few, with methodologies, measures and results which defy direct comparison.

The majority of researchers agree that generalizations based on the broad categorizations of 'congenital' versus 'acquired' have limited utility and should be resisted. As Newell and others have pointed out, those with a congenital difference will have had more opportunity to incorporate their unusual appearance into their body image, to habituate to the responses of others and to acquire effective coping strategies. However, the picture is more complex than this as some congenital conditions result in progressively more apparent differences over the life course (for example, neurofibromatosis), whereas others, although apparent at birth, are less obvious following surgical correction (for example cleft lip; craniosynostoses). Individuals who acquire a disfigurement have to deal with their feelings concerning the circumstances surrounding the onset and the loss of their previous looks while also formulating and incorporating changes to their body image. Bradbury (1997) has discussed the issues associated with an unexpected appearance change. Alterations to physical appearance can result in a profound disruption of body image for all, and for many, can constitute a major crisis. Those acquiring a visible difference as the result of a life-threatening condition such as cancer may have their appearance-related concerns suppressed or complicated by the need to undergo surgery in a bid to rid themselves of their disease. In the case of head and neck cancer, patients may also face post-surgical difficulties related to eating and speaking, together with fears of further recurrence, all of which can exacerbate or diminish appearance-related concerns.

However, even more specific categorizations such as 'skin conditions' may mask important differences. Porter et al. (1986) compared two groups of people with the skin conditions vitiligo or psoriasis with a control group. Both condition groups had lower self-esteem than controls, but those with psoriasis reported more prejudice than people with vitiligo, including being stared at and experiencing discrimination in the workplace. They also scored lower on measures of adjustment to the disorder. The researchers speculated that the increased visibility of psoriasis accounts for the greater difficulties in this group. In addition, there is mounting evidence that fluctuating conditions such as psoriasis seem to present particular difficulties in terms of the unpredictability of the visible manifestations of the condition. The reactions of others are potentially less consistent, and those affected are likely to have to be prepared to cope with a broader spectrum of responses.

Although a few studies have demonstrated differences when comparing two or three specific condition groups, Rumsey et al.'s (2004) study of levels of appearance-related distress and wellbeing in a large sample of outpatients with a wide range of visible differences showed no clear relationships between aetiology and distress. Instead, this study highlighted the extent of individual variation in adjustment within each group.

Despite widespread assumptions among the uninitiated that the aetiology and extent of a visible difference are strongly related to distress, the evidence offers a different picture. While particular conditions may present specific sets of challenges for those affected (see Chapter 4), these challenges provoke a whole range of responses rather than a predictable pattern of distress or adjustment.

*Severity, visibility and the amenability of a difference to camouflage*

It is intuitively plausible that the more severe a disfigurement, the less well adjusted the affected person will be. However, the weight of evidence indicates that objective severity is not a good predictor of levels of distress (see Moss 2005; Rumsey et al. 2004). Instead, the self-perceived severity of a disfigurement and the extent to which the affected person believes it is noticeable to others are better predictors of adjustment (Rumsey et al. 2004). Clarification of the detail of the relationship between severity and distress has been hampered by measurement difficulties (for example, defining and rating severity – see Chapter 2). Moss (2005) has recently reported that self ratings of perceived severity are significantly related to adjustment in a sample of more than 400 patients awaiting plastic and reconstructive surgery, with these ratings accounting for 20 per cent of the variance. Ratings of objective severity (completed by clinicians) suggested that severe and mild disfigurements were associated with less appearance-related distress, and moderate levels with greater distress. However, these ratings accounted for only 5 per cent of the variance.

Judgements of severity (whether objective or subjective) are likely to be affected by the extent to which a disfigurement is visible to others and many commentators have assumed that the visibility of a difference can be directly related to the stress experienced. Visible conditions affecting the face are acknowledged to be particularly distressing, especially if the eyes and mouth are affected, as these are a strong focus of attention from others during social interaction (Bull and Rumsey 1988; MacGregor 1970). If large areas of the face are affected the difference is likely to be immediately obvious in most social encounters, whereas other conditions (for example a hand injury) are less immediately visible and will become apparent in fewer situations. However, counterintuitively, several writers have noted that the impact on others of having a difference which is clearly visible is more predictable and thus easier to handle than one which is only apparent in some situations. Lansdown (1976) noted that mild disfigurements can cause as much, if not more, anxiety than highly visible conditions, as they may engender greater variability in the reactions of others. This unpredictability contributes to lack of control, resulting in raised anxiety levels. Similarly, MacGregor (1970) noted that people with obvious disfiguration experience negative reactions more consistently than those with a less noticeable difference, enabling them to develop more consistent and effective ways of coping.

Visible differences may be amenable to camouflage using make-up, prosthetics, clothes or hair. However, for some, camouflage can bring its own problems in relation to issues of self-presentation and identity ('Are people responding to the real me?'), over-reliance on the camouflaged image in social interaction and fears that the 'truth' will be discovered (see Chapter 6).

*Background appearance*

The majority of researchers have shied away from the interesting issue of the impact of background appearance on body image, and adjustment of additional appearance-related factors over and above the visible difference remains to be explored, largely because of measurement difficulties. In relation to the reactions of others, does a difference have more or less of an impact if the affected person is in other ways physically attractive than if they are not? Shaw (1981) carried out a study using photographs of children with one of five dentofacial impairments, who were judged to be attractive or unattractive. He found that the background attractiveness affected judgements of friendliness and sociability. Tobiasen and Hiebert (1993) have noted that a high level of background attractiveness can compensate for a mild visible congenital difference to give an overall appearance perceived as attractive. Intuitively, appearance factors do play a part in the equation, but this supposition needs further exploration.

And what of self-perceptions? Is the impact of a visible difference ameliorated if the affected person perceives themselves to be attractive in other ways? Starr (1980) found no differences in a sample of patients affected by a cleft. However, Newell (2000a) noted that the study suffered from various methodological weaknesses. Although the few studies in this area have related to people with differences which are discernible to others, there are signs that self-perceptions of appearance are also better predictors of distress than objective ratings of appearance in the mainsteam population (Feingold 1992). However, in view of the large range of factors which have the potential to affect adjustment, any examination of individual differences is unlikely to be explained by physical characteristics of the visible or perceived 'abnormality' in isolation, and must also include a consideration of sociocultural and psychological factors.

*Sociocultural and demographic factors*

One of the many challenges for researchers in this area is to account for any differences in how physical appearance and visible differences may be experienced and viewed by others as the result of sociocultural factors such as race, culture, gender, social class and age. One particular mountain for researchers to climb is the task of understanding and explaining differences in adjustment accounted for by ethnic group membership. A small body of research exists relating to differences between ethnic groups in relation to weight concerns (see for example, Duncan et al. 2004). However, research relating to other aspects of appearance is lacking. The few studies that exist are suggestive of sociocultural differences; for example, Rucker and Cash (1992) found that when compared with African Americans, Caucasian Americans had more negative body cognitions and evaluations of general physical appearance. In addition, Strauss (1985) has noted that in Israel, differences between western Jews, oriental Jews and Arabs exist in their explanations of the origins of congenital anomalies, and their approaches to rehabilitation and community integration. Despite an acknowledgement that this is a major gap in current understanding, the nuances of cultural and social differences in responses to visible birth anomalies, acquired differences and the appearance concerns of people drawn from more general populations remain largely uninvestigated and further research is needed.

### Age and gender

The role and interactions of developmental stage and gender in appearance-related adjustment are discussed in Chapters 3 and 4. Findings are contradictory, and although these is some support for the commonly held assumption that appearance-related distress is most common for adolescent and young adult females, evidence of high levels of distress in all age groups and for both sexes has also been demonstrated. Clear-cut conclusions are particularly difficult to achieve in relation to gender. A study by Brown et al. (1988) involving 260 burns-affected individuals hinted both at the complexity of variables involved in adjustment, and also the role of gender in this complexity. Regression analyses suggested that low functional disability, more recreational activities, greater social support, a less avoidant and a more problem-solving coping style accounted for 55 per cent of the variance in adjustment. In men the most powerful predictor was less functional disability, while for women it was the use of problem-solving coping. In a review, Newell (2000a) has also concluded that research findings examining the role of gender in adjustment to visible differences are contradictory. He also speculated that different variables are associated with better psychosocial adjustment in males compared with females.

### Socioeconomic and living status

Studies exploring any differences in levels of body dissatisfaction that may be attributable to social class are limited, and have produced conflicting results. High levels of weight concern in pupils attending schools with higher socioeconomic catchment areas have been found (Wardle and Marsland 1990); however, other studies have failed to find this effect. Robinson (1997) suggested that body shape ideals are fairly universally accessible via magazines, billboards, films and television, thus in this respect, differences between classes are likely to be minimal. Harris and Carr's (2001) study of

appearance concerns in a general population sample fo
with either socioeconomic level or living status.

Rumsey (1997) discussed the differential rates i
aesthetic surgical and orthodontic procedures to correct p
appearance. In the UK, the National Health Service will
to 'correct' all acquired disfigurements and the major
anomalies. Only in exceptional circumstances will aest
provided for those without an objective disfigurement (ᴜᴀᴛ ɪs to say, an
'abnormality' which is visible to an onlooker). In the USA, many procedures may not be covered by health insurance or national health care
schemes and the expense may be prohibitive for some. A visible disfigurement may therefore have serious financial implications for those on lower
incomes (Strauss 2001) and some interventions may therefore become only
an option for the 'elite'. The impact of the availability or rationing of treatment in different health care systems has yet to be investigated. However,
some commentators have suggested that the more widely cosmetic procedures are advertised and taken up by those who can afford them, the more
pressure is exerted to do the same both on people who are unhappy with the
way they look and also those who are more accepting of a disfigurement.

*Social support and the family environment*

The benefits of social support as a positive resource in a variety of situations
are widely accepted, and good quality social support is commonly regarded
as an asset which can be mobilized in times of crisis to act as a buffer of
stress.

Liossi (2003) found that people with appearance concerns who reported
higher levels of social support had more favourable levels of social anxiety
and social avoidance. A lower level of social support (both the number
of supportive relationships and satisfaction with support received) was a
significant predictor of appearance dissatisfaction. Her data suggested that
better quality social support may act in conjunction with more favourable
levels of self-esteem to protect people from distress even when they held
dysfunctional appearance schemata.

How might social support offer protective effects in the context of
appearance concerns? Baumeister and Leary (1995) have speculated that
social support may be helpful as it increases a person's sense of being valued.
Liossi has proposed that good social support promotes effective coping
strategies, for example, by facilitating exposure to feared situations. Personal
accounts testify to the benefits of feeling at ease with familiar others, who
are perceived as seeing through superficial appearances to the 'real' person
beneath. However, ironically, appearance concerns can limit the development and maintenance of an effective social support network, as social
avoidance and withdrawal commonly result from distress. Baker (1992)
found that positive social support improved rehabilitation outcomes for

and neck cancer patients six months after treatment. Similar findings
or children and adolescents affected by burns have been also been reported
(Blakeney et al. 1990). Orr et al. (1989) examined the effect of perceived
social support from family and friends on body image, self-esteem and
depression in adolescents and young adults affected by burns. They found
perceived support from friends to be the most critical determinant of
positive adjustment. In a study by Browne et al. (1985) those who were less
well adjusted to their burn injury perceived less support from friends, family
and peers.

Partners and families are likely to be the main providers of support for
people with appearance concerns, yet they are also often a major influence,
particularly during childhood and adolescence, in the development and
maintenance of appearance-related distress (see Chapters 3 and 4).
MacGregor and colleagues (1953) discussed the detrimental consequences
of parents placing great value on beauty and the importance of appearance
on offspring with facial disfigurements. This comment has been echoed
in the body image literature. Kearney-Cooke (2002) highlighted the
importance of affirming reactions of parents towards their children's body
shape and physical attributes, and the dangers of children internalizing a
critical approach to their own appearance. She points out that in the current
climate of normative dissatisfaction about appearance, many children are
being raised by mothers who are themselves critical and dissatisfied with
their own bodies (see Chapter 3). Smolak et al. (1999) found that verbal
criticisms from mothers were associated with body image disturbance in
adolescents and young adults, with this association stronger for females than
males.

Although specific research evidence is lacking, there is no doubt that
there is considerable variation in many child-rearing practices between
families that are likely to influence appearance-related distress or adjustment. These include the extent to which a child's worth and esteem is built
on more enduring factors than physical appearance, how each family models
their attitudes towards physical appearance (for example, the extent to
which value is attached to 'keeping up appearances' in social situations;
the emphasis on matching up to images of physical appearance portrayed in
the media) and the degree to which teasing about appearance within the
family is condoned. Similarly, families of children and teenagers with visible
differences vary greatly in the ways they deal with disfigurement. For
example, there may or may not be open discussion of the difference and any
associated problems (see Chapter 4). The way in which treatment is
approached may also be influential. How do parents present the need for
treatment to their child? How is the motivation for appearance-enhancing
treatment communicated (Hearst and Middleton 1997)?

On the basis of clinical experience, Pope (1999) feels a number of key
tasks for parents of children with congenital craniofacial differences should
be achieved to optimize adjustment. These comprise adjusting positively to

the birth of a child with a visible difference, forming strong parent–infant relationships, formulating effective ways of explaining the difference to relatives, friends and strangers, guarding against overprotection of the child, dealing with the stress associated with treatment, being accepting of the child's appearance both before and after treatment, preparing the child for new social environments such as a new school or new social group (for example, tactics for dealing with questions from classmates, how to deal with teasing, strategies for forming friendships), boosting the child's self-esteem if they are self-critical, and increasing the child/adolescent's involvement with treatment as they get older. To Pope's thoughtful list we would add the challenge for parents of all children – whether or not they have a visible difference – of ensuring that physical appearance is, at the most, only a modest determinant of self-esteem.

### The role of cognitive processes in adjustment

Although research evidence is currently lacking, many body image and appearance researchers share the assumption that a raft of cognitive processes are implicated in vulnerability and resilience to appearance concerns. For example, Liossi (2003) found evidence in qualitative interviews with young adults that a number of cognitive strategies can serve to maintain and exacerbate preoccupation with appearance. These include the tendency to be hypervigilant of the behaviour of others; making social comparisons which result in the affected person feeling inferior and inadequate; negative attributional analyses of events. For example, one participant stated that '. . . people deliberately stare to embarrass you. They say "Look at him, not one muscle in his body, he is so weak, worse than a girl" ' (p. 101).

Liossi offered examples of other cognitive distortions, including overgeneralization: 'Physically attractive people have it all . . . women, money . . . the whole world is at their feet' (p. 97), adopting a selectively negative focus, and catastrophizing. Those with high body satisfaction were characterized by accepting and valuing their physical appearance, including both differences and strong points. Societal prejudices in favour of beauty were actively challenged:

> It's unfortunate, but in today's society, people have forgotten that it's what's inside a person that counts, not what's on the outside. If we learn to love and accept ourselves, we will also begin to love our bodies, no matter what size, shape or colour we are . . .

> Women need to take a stand and stop trying to live up to the standards that society has set for us . . . diets just don't work and losing weight will never bring you true happiness.

The desirability of clarifying the role of these cognitive processes and the relationships between them is undeniable, as increased understanding would improve the chances that interventions targeted on cognitive processes could be made more effective.

## Self-esteem

Self-esteem has been defined as the self-appraisal of one's significance, worth, competence and success as compared with others (Coopersmith 1967). Liossi (2003) noted that self-esteem has been investigated in three main ways. First, as an outcome of the processes that inhibit or produce self-esteem, second, as a self-motive (the tendency for people to behave in ways that maintain or increase positive evaluations of the self) and third, as a buffer (providing protection from experiences that are harmful). All three aspects are potentially relevant to appearance research. Levels of self-esteem have been found to correlate highly with body dissatisfaction, especially for women (Ben-Tovim and Walker 1995). For men, the evidence is not so clear cut, though Mintz and Betz (1986) found a relationship for both men and women, as did Liossi (2003). There is much more to learn about the causal links between satisfaction/dissatisfaction with appearance and self-esteem. Someone who is dissatisfied with his or her appearance may extend this dissatisfaction to other aspects of the self, evaluating them more negatively and experiencing lower overall self-esteem. Alternatively, a person's positive self-esteem may result in greater satisfaction with appearance, or he/she may consider other aspects of the self to be more important determinants of self-esteem. Harter (1999) reported that teenagers who believed that appearance determined their self-worth had lower self-esteem and higher levels of depression than adolescents who believed their self-worth determined their feelings about their appearance.

In relation to buffering, some researchers (Baumeister 1997) have maintained that self-esteem works to maintain positive self-views by affecting the processing of feedback in a self-serving way. People with high self-esteem are more likely than those with low self-esteem to perceive appearance-related (and other) feedback as consistent with their positive self-views, to work to discredit the source of negative feedback, and to access other important aspects of the self to counteract the negative views. Others (Liossi 2003) argue that people with high self-esteem have a more stable sense of self and are less emotionally labile than people with low self-esteem. Both of these elements contribute to a kind of stable emotional anchor with which to weather life's challenges. It has also been suggested that people with higher self-esteem have more adaptive 'cognitive resources' at their disposal which enable them to deal more effectively with difficult circumstances and external pressures. Grogan (1999) suggested that a favourable body-image is linked with positive feelings about the self together with feelings of self-confidence and power in social situations. Several of the participants in Liossi's study talked of personal agency in the way appearance information is handled: 'The diet and fashion industries are not totally to blame for society's obsession with thinness. We are the ones keeping them in business . . . We buy their magazines, diet books and gym equipment' (2003: 105).

*Levels of investment in appearance*

Some researchers believe that an understanding of the appearance-related components of self-perceptions is crucial to clarifying why some people are more prone to appearance distress than others. Current interest surrounds the relative salience of appearance within the self-concept and the extent to which a person evaluates their appearance positively or negatively (valence; see Chapter 2). Appearance may also be judged by individuals as being closer to, or further from their internalized cultural ideals (Altabe and Thompson 1996). The appearance aspect of the self-representation can be more or less salient at any time, playing a greater or lesser part in the work-ing self-concept (Higgins and Brendl 1995). There will therefore be vari-ation in the extent to which a person's perception of his/her appearance is involved in attending to and appraising activity in the social environment, and in interpreting subsequent memories of social encounters (Moss and Carr 2004). Theorists speculate that when appearance is generally more salient, negatively valenced, and further from ideals, adjustment is likely to be poorer. Some of the important ways in which appearance might become more salient and prone to negative evaluation include positive or negative experiences of social encounters (see Chapters 3 and 4), subjective percep-tions of the perceived severity and the perceived noticeability of a visible difference to others, and social comparison processes (Green and Sedikides 2001).

In the attempt to further explain individual differences in body satisfac-tion or dissatisfaction, some researchers, most notably Cash (1996; Cash et al. 2004) have taken the concepts of salience and valence one step further. They have proposed the existence of appearance-related cognitive schemata which result in attentional sensitivity to comments about one's appearance, and interpretative biases in processing feedback from others. Markus (1977) described self-schemas as 'cognitive generalisations about the self, derived from past experience, that organise and guide the processing of self-related information contained in the individual's social experiences'. Schemas are comprised of both structure (the associative networks) and content (beliefs or principles). People are said to be schematic on a particular dimension if they regard the dimension as a central and salient feature of their self-concept, and aschematic if they do not. Thus, if a child's appearance is the focus of negative criticism, he or she will begin to develop a schema with the negative aspect as a feature. With repetition the person becomes faster and more efficient at seeing themselves as unacceptable, and this becomes an automatic thought in response to a variety of situations. Pathology can also develop and be maintained through the types of information that comprise the schema (for example, dysfunctional attitudes and negative automatic thoughts), the way it is organized (for example, the strength of the connections between informational nodes) and the way information is processed within the schema (for example, using overgeneralization, selective abstraction and so on).

In Cash's (1996) cognitive-behavioural model of body dissatisfaction he proposes that people have schemas about physical appearance derived from past experience and influenced by personality and physical attributes. Environmental stimuli about appearance from any number of sources can activate this appearance-related or body image schema, which in turn, influence affect and behaviour. In people with such a schema, Cash and Labarge (1996) believe that self-esteem is closely tied to feelings about physical appearance. Research findings have largely supported the various components of Cash's model, although a comprehensive testing of the whole package of processes remains a challenge (see Chapter 2). In research investigating the interpretations of appearance and health-related sentences by weight-preoccupied and asymptomatic women, Jackman et al. (1995) found that weight-preoccupied women showed an information processing bias that was consistent with their negative view of their body. Similar results have been found by Cooper (1997) in the interpretations of ambiguous interpersonal situations; by Tantleff-Dunn and Thompson (1998) in the selective attention and recall of information; and by Wood et al. (1998) and Altabe and Thompson (1996) in the completion of ambiguous appearance and non-appearance-related sentences. Liossi (2003) found people concerned with appearance had higher levels of appearance schematicity and psychological distress, and lower levels of self-esteem and social support than people who were not concerned about their appearance. The existence of appearance schemata was the most significant predictor of appearance dissatisfaction in her regression analyses. The results showed that young adults placing more cognitive importance on appearance (they were high in appearance schematicity) were more vulnerable to negative feelings, had lower self-esteem, experienced more psychological distress and more dissatisfaction with their appearance. Her findings are consistent with those of cognitive theorists (for example, Cooper 1997) who maintain that the content of dysfunctional appearance-related attitudes includes the belief that appearance determines personal worth.

*Comparisons with others*

Another group of processes that has received attention from writers interested in adjustment, appearance and visible difference is that of social comparison. Social Comparison Theory (Festinger 1954) claimed that we engage in relatively continuous comparisons of our characteristics, strengths and weaknesses with others so that we can ascertain our relative standing in our social environment. The process is spontaneous, effortless, unintentional and common, and the need to know how one is doing in comparison with others increases significantly at times of stress as uncertainty is uncomfortable. Downward (favourable) comparisons involve comparisons between the self and others who are worse off ('I have lost part of my face because of cancer, but I'm better off than others I have seen in the clinic'). Upward (unfavourable) comparisons with others who are perceived as being better off tend to be less adaptive. For example, studies provide convincing evidence that media images play a significant role in how women feel about their bodies (Grogan 1999), and if people pick the idealized appearance of models, film or TV idols as relevant reference points for comparison this is likely to result in greater dissatisfaction with their own appearance.

Researchers have identified differences both in the extent to which people engage in social comparison and in their tendency to favour upward or downward comparisons. In a study by Gibbons (1999), participants' reports of the extent to which they engaged in downward comparison were positively correlated with their reports of positive affect or wellbeing. Stormer and Thompson (1996) found in a sample of 162 college students that the frequency of appearance comparisons explained more variance in levels of body satisfaction than other potential predictors including teasing history and levels of internalization of sociocultural pressures relating to attractiveness, with the frequency of comparisons accounting for 32 per cent of the variance after self-esteem and body mass were covaried. Beebe et al. (1996) found that women who place a strong emphasis on their own appearance concerns also assume that others are preoccupied with similar issues and emphasize these when evaluating others. They are likely to engage in more social comparisons than their less preoccupied counterparts, and to rate the social comparisons as important to their own self-evaluations. These findings suggest that differences in the way people engage in the process of social comparison may explain some of the variation in satisfaction and dissatisfaction with appearance. Thompson (2004) has noted that more needs to be learned, particularly about the effects of frequent upward comparisons on adjustment.

*Optimism*

In health psychology, the current consensus is that optimism is adaptive in the face of adversity – for example, people with an optimistic explanatory style are less likely to develop physical ill health or depression when they face major events (Carr 2004). Although research specifically examining optimism in the context of appearance is currently lacking, anecdotal reports from commentators on adjustment following disfigurement have suggested that people with an optimistic outlook on life deal better with the consequences of a difference which is visible to others. An additional attraction of promoting research in this area is that some researchers believe that optimism can be taught – for example, Seligman (1998) has developed programmes to help adults and children change from a pessimistic to an optimistic view on life. Therefore, although the jury is still out in relation to specific links between optimism and appearance-related adjustment, there would appear to be enough evidence from relevant fields to suggest this construct should remain on the shortlist of factors that may promote resilience and may in part explain individual differences in adjustment.

*Coping styles*

Adaptive and maladaptive coping styles have been investigated in relation to the body image concerns and adjustment of people with disfigurements, though much of the evidence is anecdotal (see Moss (1997) for an overview). Until recently, it has been assumed that the use of denial or an avoidant coping style are inadvisable in the context of disfigurement, as these were thought to further exacerbate fears relating to a particular situation and to postpone the development of more effective strategies. However, Pillemer and Cook (1989) suggested that for some children with facial differences, denial might act as a defence mechanism in order to protect their self-esteem. Robinson et al. (1996) and others have noted that avoidance (for example, of a potentially embarrassing situation) can also be helpful as one of a more extensive repertoire of coping strategies. They suggested that rather than eliminate particular supposedly maladaptive coping strategies, interventions should focus on broadening the number and variety of coping skills a person has at their disposal, with a view to increasing the flexibility with which those affected can respond both to variations in their own mood, and to the varied and often unpredictable demands of social situations.

Despite this scepticism about the utility of pronouncing particular coping styles to be more or less adaptive, some useful insights continue to be generated by the coping literature. A four-item sub-scale of the COPE measuring 'positive reinterpretation and growth' was used by Fortune et al. (2005) in a prospective study of 95 people with psoriasis which was designed to explore the predictors of a construct termed 'adversarial growth', defined as the ability to construe benefits resulting from negative events. At six-month follow-up, 18 per cent of the sample were identified as displaying signs of this construct. The authors reported that this group of participants was characterized by their relative youth at the time of onset of psoriasis and the realism of their beliefs about the condition (in particular the acknowledgement that the condition is chronic, recurring and essentially incurable). In accordance with the weight of recent research evidence, the clinical severity of the condition was not a strong predictor, neither were measures of anxiety or depression, gender or socioeconomic status. Once

again the evidence points to the key role of ɑ
and distress.

*The role of social interaction skills*

Many of the difficulties experienced f
centre on the intricacies of social inte'
those affected has therefore been the fo
Fear of negative evaluation by othe'
appear to have a central role in social ɑ.
body image, regardless of the actual behaviour of ou.
effective social skills involve an element of taking respoi.
behaviour and reactions of others.

Partridge (1990: 123) explained that 'you will be scrutinised and automatic assumptions will be made in the public's mind, about your looks and
your character. These connections are rarely flattering and will persist unless
you challenge them'.

Persuasive arguments have been put forward that good social skills result
in more positive experiences of social interaction and in better adjustment
among people with visible differences (Rumsey et al. 1986; see also Chapter
4). Partridge (personal communication) described how he changed from
being self-conscious and scared after his burn injury to being more self-
assured;

> I discovered that provided I had a strong and positive attitude . . . a
> very big IF . . . I could manipulate by my behaviour how people
> responded to me, especially in the first crucial moments of a meeting.
> I experimented with different levels of eye-contact, handshake, verbal
> energy and body language, and eventually mastered encounters with
> others.

Researchers have also demonstrated the beneficial effects of social interaction skills training for people with visible differences (Kapp-Simon et al.
1992; Robinson et al. 1996; Rumsey et al. 1986). The potential benefits of
similar interventions for people debilitated by other appearance concerns
remain to be explored. However, promising results from similar approaches
used to tackle the social avoidance and negative self-perceptions of people
suffering from shyness have been reported by Crozier (2001).

## Conclusion

Researchers have recently begun to devote their energies to clarifying the
factors and processes which contribute to resilience or exacerbate distress in
relation to appearance. This chapter has assembled current thinking relating
to the most likely suspects in relation to adjustment. However, the belief or

...t there are a limited number of straightforward relation-
... a few variables is naïve and even potentially misleading.
...al questions of cause and effect and the relative contribution
...rious factors to adjustment remain unanswered. The cognitive
...es linking upbringing, past experience, self-image, beliefs about
... others think about us and the perceived reactions of others are
...gely complex and mind-blowing in their circularity. Complete clarity
...oncerning the processes involved remains a distant promise, but the
journey is likely to be illuminating, not just for appearance researchers, but
also those with a broader interest in the components of adjustment and
wellbeing.

## Chapter summary

- Most research has focused on the difficulties associated with visible difference and appearance concerns, but individual differences are considerable, and some people adjust positively;
- In contrast to the earlier emphasis on the problems associated with disfigurement, researchers are now devoting more effort to identifying factors associated with positive coping, with a view to using the information to inform interventions;
- The physical characteristics of a disfigurement (aetiology, severity) play a relatively minor role in adjustment, though visibility can exacerbate problems;
- Little part is played in adjustment by demographic differences. However, more needs to be learned about the influence of a person's cultural context;
- Appearance is a more salient aspect of self-esteem for some, and can dominate social information processing;
- Those with high levels of body dissatisfaction tend to engage in more upward comparisons with inappropriate targets of comparison;
- Good quality social support and social skills appear to contribute to positive adjustment;
- Appearance-related adjustment is multifactorial. Although some contributory factors have been identified, the interrelationships and relative weight of the factors involved remain to be clarified.

## Discussion points

- How would you define resilience?
- How might resilience to appearance concerns be promoted or taught?
- How much importance did your family attach to outward appearances?
- How much impact does your appearance have on your self-esteem?

♦ How might you tease out the various cognitive components of adjustment in relation to appearance?

## Further reading

Cash, T.F. (2002b) Cognitive-behavioral perspectives on body image, in T.F. Cash
and T. Pruzinsky (eds) *Body Image: A Handbook of Theory, Research and Clinical
Practice*. London: The Guilford Press.
Partridge, J. (1990) *Changing Faces*. London: Penguin.

# CHAPTER 6

# Current provision of support and intervention for appearance-related concerns

*(with contributions from Alex Clarke)*

Previous chapters have highlighted the nature of appearance-related concerns among people with or without a visible difference and shown that they can usefully be seen as a continuum for the whole population. But how are these issues addressed and what sources of support and interventions are available for individuals with these concerns? We now critically consider the current provision of support and interventions in the UK. In Chapter 7 we permit ourselves the luxury of an 'ideal world' and suggest how care might best be delivered.

This chapter starts by considering ways in which the majority of individuals seek to deal with any dissatisfaction with their appearance, either by changing their physical looks, the emphasis they give to it or the cognitive processes by which they appraise and evaluate their appearance. We then consider the limited sources of support available within the community, highlight the increasing popularity of 'quick fix' interventions such as cosmetic surgical or non-surgical procedures and examine their effectiveness in addressing appearance concerns. We then focus on the care and support for people with a visible difference provided through self-help groups and charitable organizations and biomedical treatments provided through health care services. Having highlighted the strengths and limitations of a biomedical framework, we examine the potential benefits of using a biopsychosocial approach in this context.

## Support and intervention for the population as a whole

In marked contrast to the appreciation of appearance-related distress among people with a visible difference, there has been a tendency not to recognize the extent and debilitating impact of appearance concerns in the general population (see Chapter 3). Notable exceptions are the professional care and support for individuals who, at the more extreme end of the appearance concern continuum have been diagnosed as having eating disorders or body dysmorphic disorder (in which an affected individual imagines or grossly exaggerates a visible difference). Readers are directed towards Phillips (2002) and Veale (2004) for recent excellent reviews of body dysmorphic disorder.

### Self-management of appearance

While many people report being dissatisfied with their appearance, the majority do not seek or receive any professional help or support in this respect. Most people find their own ways of managing any discordance between their perceived actual and ideal appearance, for example by investing their time and money in beauty products, clothing, hairstyles and exercise regimes (see Chapter 1). While some such activities have clear health benefits (for example maintaining a healthy diet) others can be detrimental to health (for example exposure to the sun or using anabolic steroids). In essence individuals engaging in these behaviours are seeking to alter the objective information that informs self-appraisal of appearance (they are trying to alter their physical appearance). These activities might be the limit of an individual's attempts to change or control their appearance and for many they are enjoyable, sometimes social activities.

Yet others, in addition to (or instead of) focusing on their physical, objective appearance, attempt to reconcile any dissonance by altering their thoughts, appraisals and beliefs about their looks. In effect, they engage in cognitive processes to alter the value and importance they place on appearance or the comparisons they make between themselves and others (this relates to the framework suggested in Chapter 2 and processes outlined in Chapter 5). An array of resources are available to help them in this process, including self-help materials such as Cash's *Body Image Workbook* (1997) (see Box 6.1).

While research has demonstrated that self-directed cognitive-behavioural programmes can be as efficient as therapist-led interventions (see Cash and Strachan 2002), most self-help resources have not been systematically evaluated and tend to focus solely on attitudes towards body size and weight.

Some individuals seek further support and intervention, for example through organizations in the community, by visiting their general practitioner (GP) or seeking cosmetic surgical and non-surgical interventions. Although this chapter considers these various avenues as discrete options, in reality individuals may simultaneously engage in a variety of activities and be influenced by a multitude of factors including significant others and the media.

---

**Box 6.1   The Body Image Workbook**

This is an eight-stage programme based on cognitive-behavioural principles involving:

♦ self-assessment of influences upon body image
♦ recording body image experiences
♦ relaxation training and desensitization
♦ identifying and challenging appearance assumptions
♦ cognitive restructuring
♦ replacing maladaptive with adaptive behaviours and coping strategies
♦ developing exercises to increase positive, pleasurable experiences and relationships with the body
♦ maintaining change and preventing relapse.

Developed from a body image therapy programme intended for use by professionals, this self-help format involving a workbook and minimal professional contact and encouragement through scheduled telephone calls has been shown to reduce investment in appearance and increase body satisfaction (Cash and Lavallee 1997).

---

*Self-help and voluntary support groups*

In contrast to the number of support organizations available for people with a disfigurement there is a dearth of community-based and voluntary support for individuals who do not have a visible difference but who are troubled by concerns about their appearance. A notable exception is the widespread availability of support for people whose concerns revolve around their weight. Slimming clubs such as Weight Watchers offer advice and guidance about dieting but, crucially, they also provide social support and the chance to meet others in a similar situation. Clearly this is an extremely popular approach: according to the organization's own figures, more than 6000 Weight Watcher meetings take place every week in the UK alone. In 2002 a charitable organization, Weight Concern was established in response to growing concern over obesity rates in the UK and the distress and prejudice experienced by people affected. Its aims include providing a forum for overweight people to express their views and educating health care professionals and the public about the causes of obesity and management of obese people. It has also been involved in the development and evaluation of treatment programmes for overweight children and adults. Meanwhile, self-help and voluntary support groups exist for those with eating disorders but other appearance-related concerns among people without a visible difference are unlikely to be catered for in this way.

*Support through primary care*

Patients may present to primary care services with a range of physical and psychosocial problems which may be directly or indirectly related to appearance and related concerns. Indeed a significant proportion of GP consultations are thought to relate to dermatological conditions alone (Papadopoulos and Bor 1999). Some individuals may be referred on to specialist services while others may be prescribed treatment at this level or dismissed as not needing intervention. Services for people whose appearance concerns do not meet criteria for NHS treatment might be limited to information and advice regarding appropriate self-management such as diet and exercise. Interestingly, while current UK Government policy (Department of Health 2004) prioritizes attention and primary care resources towards the increasing rates of obesity on the grounds of associated health concerns, it may be concerns about appearance that encourage overweight individuals to seek help or engage in weight-reducing behaviours.

*Cosmetic surgical and non-surgical intervention*

Some aspects of appearance, such as the shape of one's nose, will not change without surgical intervention but do not meet criteria for plastic or reconstructive surgery (in the UK a very limited range of procedures are freely available on the NHS). Increasingly, individuals who are unhappy with their appearance but do not match NHS criteria are seeking private cosmetic interventions. Those who have sought help elsewhere may believe a cosmetic surgery consultation is the only situation in which their concerns are taken seriously. Cosmetic interventions may be appealing because the results are hopefully achieved quickly and relatively easily – having made the decision, the role of the individual is one of passivity. In contrast, changing body shape via exercise or diet is likely to be a slow, arduous process requiring ongoing will-power and commitment.

It has been suggested (Pertschuk et al. 1998) that the profile of people seeking private cosmetic treatments has changed over recent years so that they are no longer seen as exclusive treatments for the elite and wealthy (Sarwer 2002). Yet the cost involved still renders cosmetic surgery an 'unnecessary' expense and a luxury item for many. Sarwer and Crerand (2004) cite direct marketing, media coverage and the availability of less-invasive and safer procedures as factors in the increased acceptance and take-up of surgical and non-surgical cosmetic procedures (see Box 6.2).

The number of people willing to undergo the inherent risks of surgical or non-surgical treatments in the absence of illness or disease can be considered a testimony to the desire to alter their appearance, often permanently. Kathy Davis (1995) argues that the increase in the number of women undergoing cosmetic surgery is a sign that they are taking charge of their

---

**Box 6.2    Recent trends in cosmetic procedures**

♦ The American Society of Plastic Surgeons (ASPS) (cited in Sarwer and Crerand 2004) report that the number of Americans undergoing cosmetic surgical and non-surgical treatments increased by 1600 per cent in the ten-year period prior to 2002;

♦ The British Association of Aesthetic Plastic Surgeons (BAAPS) calculated that more than 21,000 private cosmetic procedures were performed in 2002 in the UK. However, this is a conservative figure since membership of the society is not compulsory;

♦ Non-surgical cosmetic procedures (such as Botox treatment and chemical peels) now surpass surgical procedures in the USA (ASPS 2003, cited in Sarwer and Crerand 2004). According to the ASPS, 92,000 Americans underwent chemical skin peels in 2002, compared with 19,000 in 1992. BAAPS estimates that more than 75,000 Botox injections were given in the UK in 2002;

♦ According to BAAPS the number of men undergoing cosmetic surgical procedures in the UK increased by 60 per cent between 2003 and 2004.

---

lives and maximizing their chances in a culture that privileges the attractive. Interestingly, while some people who elect cosmetic treatment are willing for this to become public knowledge, many do not want others to know that they have ventured down this path. This may be because their aim (like that of many people with a visible difference) is to look 'ordinary' as opposed to 'extraordinary' and not to stand out, or because they fear accusations of vanity. It has been suggested that individuals seeking treatment for what could be considered an 'aesthetic' disfigurement could be encouraged to accept their appearance rather than undergo cosmetic surgery (Oberle and Allen 1994); however, it seems realistic to assume that the demand for such procedures will continue.

Sarwer et al. (1997: 1) claim that 'cosmetic surgery can be considered a psychological intervention, or at a minimum, a surgical procedure with psychological consequences'. A body of literature has emerged regarding individuals' motivations, experiences and satisfaction with cosmetic treatments. This research shows that such interventions are often effective in improving self-reported body image and satisfaction with the part of the body that has received treatment, without increasing dissatisfaction with the rest of the body (Sarwer 2002; Sarwer and Crerand 2004). However, there is a lack of research examining the longer-term impact of cosmetic procedures so it is unclear whether the perceived benefits of treatment are maintained once the early 'euphoria' of a changed appearance has worn off. Similarly, research has yet to examine the psychological issues around electing to undergo non-surgical (for example botox treatment) as opposed to surgical procedures, although Sarwer and Crerand (2004) suggest that Sarwer's model of cosmetic surgery and body image (see Chapter 2) applies equally well to both types of procedure.

As increasing numbers of people undergo these treatments it is inevitable that more and more will experience failed procedures and side-effects. In such circumstances the possibility for regret and recrimination is high, as individuals may blame themselves for having undergone 'unnecessary' surgery. Although he fails to give supporting evidence, Hughes (1998) suggests that a growing number of individuals who have undergone cosmetic surgery are seeking plastic surgery through the NHS in order to 'correct' or 'improve' the results of earlier treatment. While failed cosmetic procedures appeal to the sensationalist side of the media, there is a noticeable dearth of research into the psychosocial impact of such experiences. However, an enhanced awareness of such issues could enable the provision of appropriate support for those in this situation and is also needed if individuals are to give truly informed consent before undergoing such procedures. Exceptionally, a very small literature has emerged in relation to the experiences of women who have had breast implants removed (a process known as explantation). According to figures produced by the American Society of Plastic Surgeons (cited in Sarwer and Crerand 2004) more than 43,000 women underwent implant explantation in the USA in 2002 compared with 32,000 in 1998. The latest figures available in the UK from the National Breast Implant Registry (2004) indicate that just over 10,000 women underwent breast implant surgery in 2002. This figure included 1414 patients undergoing implant replacement procedures and 79 women who underwent implant explantation without having the implants replaced. However, these figures may not represent the full picture since registration of implants is voluntary in the UK. Walden et al. (1997) suggest that the impact on the individual can be dramatic and similar to that of losing a breast due to cancer treatment. Worryingly, the vast majority of women who have breast implants are likely to be in this situation at some stage since they typically need to be replaced approximately every ten years. Further research is needed in this area.

It is important to remember that these attempts at altering physical appearance (including cosmetic surgery) or changing appearance-related beliefs and appraisals are not the sole preserve of people without a visible difference. People who have a disfigurement affecting one part of their body might still seek to alter other aspects of their appearance. This is clearly demonstrated in Marc Crank's description of his experiences of living with neurofibromatosis: 'I know what I dislike about my face and that may not be the most "abnormal" thing about it. It can be quite a task persuading a surgeon that "I know the skin on my forehead is scarred but I don't care; what I really want is my ear moving two centimetres!" ' (Lansdown et al. 1997.)

## Support and intervention for people with a visible difference

### Support through the community and voluntary sector

Much of the support for people with concerns relating to a visible difference is provided by the voluntary sector through lay-led, charitable organizations such as Changing Faces and Let's Face It, and condition-specific support groups. The famous Guinea Pig Club whose members underwent pioneering plastic and reconstructive surgery during the Second World War was probably the first appearance-related self-help group. Such organizations typically offer information and one-to-one or group support. Support for children and adolescents who have a visible difference, typically as a result of burn injuries or cancer, is increasingly available through camps, similar to summer camps in the USA.

Support groups can offer a range of benefits. First, this may be an individual's first opportunity to meet others with similar appearance issues. Importantly, this can provide the opportunity to express feelings and concerns with people who are independent of family or friends who themselves may be distressed by the situation. Second, they are an opportunity to share experiences of coping strategies found to be more or less effective. These can be practical (for example, offering advice on how to use camouflage make-up) or emotional (for example, offering support). Importantly, such groups provide the opportunity for ongoing support beyond the hospital environment and the acute phase of treatment. They may also offer support for family and friends and many provide social events in a supportive environment that may be especially valuable for those who are anxious about social situations (see Partridge and Nash (1997) for a fuller discussion). Clearly there is much demand for such groups and their success is demonstrated by their continued growth – Let's Face It was originally established in the UK and now has groups in the USA, Australia, Norway and India (Piff 1998).

However, while some people flourish in a support group, others do not and will actively avoid them for fear of being seen as a member of a group perceived as stigmatized in some way (Rumsey and Harcourt 2004). Approaching and joining a group can be a daunting experience, especially if an individual fears being judged by their appearance and has had previous negative experiences of meeting new people. Partridge and Robinson (1995) outlined potential problems with burns support groups. Specifically, an individual might compare their own appearance with that of other members of the group and be shocked to think that they themselves might have a similar appearance either now or in the future. Moreover, there is a danger that groups could focus on negative experiences and thereby become a 'wallowing' rather than therapeutic experience. There is also a possibility that group members will be adversely affected by the negative experiences of other members, for example disappointment surrounding the outcome of longed-for treatment.

Finally, the motivation of patients and individuals offering their support to groups must be clearly understood to avoid any possible detrimental impact upon either them or the group participants. Professionals and family and friends might feel torn between offering support while not wanting members to become overly dependent on them (see Partridge and Nash (1997) and Hughes (1998) for further consideration of the possible limitations of help groups). There is also a danger that rather than promoting diversity of appearance, a condition-specific group may actually promote segregation.

Unfortunately the work of support groups or individuals providing support (including camps and the general work by clinicians and health care professionals) is often not evaluated (Strauss and Broder 1991). Clear evidence of their success would be beneficial when identifying areas for improvement and change. Exceptionally, Cooper and Burnside (1996) reported a retrospective survey of an adult burns support group. Individuals tended to join a group after having one-to-one sessions that helped them to prepare for group participation. Importantly, the group aimed to be flexible in reacting to the needs of the group members and was seen as integral to standard care for burn-injured people, making it easier for patients to accept. Individuals valued the availability and flexibility of a group as a resource they could call upon any time after their burn injury, not just in the early post-trauma period. They also valued staff leading these groups, while elsewhere (Wallace and Lees 1988) participants have preferred groups to be run by their members without staff being present. This raises the interesting question 'Can individuals without a disfigurement facilitate a group for those who do?' Ultimately the skills of the facilitator (not their appearance) may determine the success and longevity of a group.

However, a group is not necessarily the most appropriate means of addressing all concerns and Cooper and Burnside's (1996) evaluation found that participants preferred sensitive issues such as sex and bereavement to be discussed in more personal, individual sessions. In contrast, Maddern and Owen (2004) point out that group sessions are preferable for some since they can find the notion of individual sessions rather uncomfortable. The organization Changing Faces offers a workshop on intimacy for adult clients with concerns about personal or intimate relationships. This workshop includes sessions on body language and communication skills, discussing appearance and anticipating others' needs. Again, this format will not suit everyone and it seems eminently sensible for psychosocial support to be made available in a variety of formats.

Support groups can offer benefits to many individuals but are best provided as part of a comprehensive package of support. While groups and organizations may encourage an individual to alter their attitude towards their appearance and lend invaluable support in dealing with others' reactions, people who are troubled by a visible difference may still seek to alter their physical appearance by way of the alternatives provided within the health care system.

*Intervention through health care services*

*Primary care*

In the UK, health care services (for example specialist treatment centres and consultants) providing the interventions outlined in this section are usually accessed via general practitioners (GPs) who therefore have a key role to play in the provision of care and act as 'gatekeepers' to specialist services. One-third of the referrals to a specialist support service for people with a visible difference reported by Kleve et al. (2002) were made by a GP, suggesting that those in the surrounding geographical area were aware of the need and availability of such support. However, since specialist support services are not widely available it is unclear how GPs in other areas deal with appearance issues. Research (Broomfield et al. 1997) suggests that patients do not feel their support needs are met through the primary care sector, indicating the potential for much improvement.

Charlton et al. (2003) called for GPs to explore patients' ideas, concerns and expectations in order to reach a shared understanding of their disfigurement and any anticipated changes in appearance. GPs need a good understanding of body image dissatisfaction, possible effects on social functioning and effective methods of support and intervention, but there is a danger that appearance-related issues might be overlooked or trivialized by health care professionals including GPs. This may not be deliberate, but could reflect a lack of confidence in recognizing and dealing with psychosocial and appearance concerns. Despite the number of people who have some kind of visible difference, a GP might only care for two or three patients with a severe facial disfigurement (Clarke 1999). However, this does not diminish the need for them to have an awareness of appearance issues, since they are likely to have very many patients without a visible difference who still have significant appearance-related distress.

McGrouther (1997) highlighted the potential role that GPs could play in the provision of care for people with appearance-related concerns. He suggested they would be more successful in assessing the personal impact of disfigurement than would a specialist who could only rely on a brief consultation as opposed to a long-standing relationship and association with the patient. However, the reality is that such an idealized doctor–patient relationship may have fallen victim to pressured GP consultations and the move towards group primary care practices. This means that continuity of a relationship is not guaranteed, as patients may see one of a number of GPs, each of whom will have their own value judgements about the importance of appearance and treatment. They may also have limited knowledge of, or contact with patients with particular appearance concerns, compared with a consultant whose specialty includes a majority of patients with visible differences. Fortunately, psychosocial issues are receiving increasing attention at specialist conferences and within relevant journals and we are therefore hopeful that at a minimum, specialist consultants might have greater awareness of the possible psychological implications of the condition they treat. However, data from our own research (Rumsey et al. 2004) suggest that this is not currently the case or perhaps that awareness does not necessarily translate into practice.

Reasons for failing to discuss or address appearance-related issues within primary care include the pressure on limited resources such as staff time and physical space (see Bradbury and Middleton 1997). Adequate time and privacy are needed in busy health care settings including GP surgeries and outpatient departments in order to facilitate discussion of sensitive and personal issues, including those relating to appearance. GP surgeries can be a useful and readily identifiable location for resources including self-help literature and information for patients, their families and carers but clearly the provision of psychosocial care and support in this setting warrants further research and clinical attention.

*Medical and surgical interventions*

Without doubt, the primary goals of treatment following trauma or diagnosis of disease must be to preserve life, restore vital function and contain the spread of disease, as appropriate. Developments in surgical and medical treatments provided through secondary and tertiary services mean that many people who would previously have been considered 'untreatable or inoperable' may now undergo biomedical interventions that may themselves result in obvious scarring or disfigurement. For example patients treated for major burns or cancer may be offered radical surgery with a resultant loss of function and altered appearance. While offering many benefits, not least saving lives, such treatment may substitute one 'condition' or 'problem' with another.

Beyond this first stage, and for people with a congenital condition such as a port wine stain that alters appearance rather than function, the aims of treatment (including surgery, drug regimes and laser treatment) are aesthetic and often involve multiple procedures over an extended period of time. This could include the possibility of 'tidying up' or 'refining' scars, which can be alluring to the patient who is dissatisfied with the aesthetic outcome of previous treatment.

*Reconstructive and plastic surgery*

Reconstructive procedures aim to restore the shape or apparent presence of a feature and include an array of techniques including transfer of skin and tissue from one part of the patient's body to another, the expansion of existing tissue in order to increase the amount of useable skin and the use of implants. They cannot recreate the original feature or restore function. Plastic surgery techniques involve modifying existing tissue and include liposuction, augmentation and surgery for ears and nose (readers are referred to Harris (1997) for an overview of limitations of plastic and reconstructive procedures).

Expectations of the outcome of plastic or reconstructive surgery may be especially high and their effects on body image are complex, involving physical, psychological and social variables (Pruzinsky 2002). Over recent years these procedures have become increasingly available within the NHS in the UK. In 2002–1 more than 15,000 patients in England underwent reconstructive surgery of some kind and they are now standard care for many patients, on the basis that they offer benefits in terms of improved quality of life and body image. For example, NHS policy (NHS Executive 1996) dictates that reconstructive breast surgery must be available to all women who undergo mastectomy for treatment of breast cancer.

While decision making about any treatment can be difficult, making choices about appearance-altering treatment such as plastic and reconstructive surgery can be especially stressful because the aesthetic outcome is uncertain. For example, the extent to which scars will be keloid (raised or coloured) after treatment is difficult to predict, even if the individual has previous scarring with which comparisons could be made. These procedures are not without the potential risks of any surgical treatment and while they aspire to improve the appearance of one part of the body, this may be at the cost of incurring new scarring on another site from where donor tissue has been removed. These 'trade offs' must be clearly explained to potential patients in order that they have reasonable expectations and can make fully informed choices. These interventions require major commitment from the patient since they are typically complicated procedures and can involve several operations before an acceptable result is obtained. Furthermore, difficult and complex decisions might be made in particularly traumatic circumstances, such as soon after a diagnosis has been made, an accident has taken place or during an ongoing series of painful procedures. For example, the possibility of reconstructive surgery is usually presented around the time of diagnosis of breast cancer and can involve a variety of options regarding the timing (immediate or delayed) and type of procedure to be undertaken. Harcourt and Rumsey (2004) found that many patients chose to put decisions about breast reconstruction 'on hold' until they were aware of the success or otherwise of their primary cancer treatment. Several also reported feeling overloaded and incapable of making complex decisions about their future physical appearance in the midst of such emotional circumstances.

The widely assumed psychological benefits of such surgery are largely unsupported by sound research evidence (see Harcourt and Rumsey 2001; NHS Executive 1996). Prospective research (Harcourt and Rumsey 2004) has found that while reconstructive breast surgery is helpful and beneficial to many women, many have to contend with persistent discomfort and extensive scarring as a result of the surgery. This was often seen as 'the price to be paid' for treatment of the disease and restored looks. In the meantime, levels of distress and changes in body image satisfaction did not differ significantly between those who had elected for or against reconstructive surgery, suggesting it is not necessarily a panacea for the distress caused by mastectomy (Harcourt et al. 2003).

The question of when reconstructive surgery is essentially purely a cosmetic procedure stimulates considerable debate and controversy. Cosmetic surgery is explicitly rationed within the NHS, yet debate persists as to whether or not, given their psychological benefits, some procedures such as tattoo removal or breast reduction, should be made more or less readily available (Horlock et al. 1999; Klassen et al. 1996). National guidelines for the provision of reconstructive procedures within the NHS in the UK are currently being developed since there are insufficient resources to meet demand and existing policy appears to vary from region to region. Ultimately, since decisions on the availability of plastic and reconstructive surgery within the NHS are still based within the biomedical framework, procedures may be sanctioned in terms of functional as opposed to psychological issues. For example, breast reduction surgery might be justified in terms of shoulder and back pain, whereas breast augmentation procedures are harder to justify on a solely functional basis. Yet both situations can have an equally devastating impact on social anxiety, self-consciousness, quality of life and sexual behaviour and both procedures have been found highly effective in terms of outcome and patient satisfaction (see Shakespeare and Cole 1997; Young et al. 1994). The decision to limit procedures such as these, which have demonstrated positive psychological outcomes, can be frustrating given the routine availability of procedures that have less favourable outcomes (for example, the general revision of scarring).

Using a framework that bases rationing on the likelihood that the procedure will impact on the problem (be that psychosocial or physical) is more logical than basing decisions on aetiology. Similarly, it is inappropriate to prioritize or ration the availability of a particular procedure on the basis of an objective assessment of the extent of disfigurement since this precludes treatment for those who experience greater psychological distress related to a less extensive or severe disfigurement (see Chapter 5). If services are allocated on the basis of perceived psychological need then this may encourage the use of self-report measures as screening tools. The problem is that those seeking surgery could easily give the responses that increase the likelihood of treatment since the wording of these measures (for example the Derriford Appearance Scale; GHQ) is typically such that it is clearly evident which responses would denote increased distress (see Chapter 2).

Finally, the ongoing developments in cosmetic and reconstructive procedures raise a plethora of ethical and moral dilemmas, plus questions regarding the psychosocial aspects of such advances, for example facial transplantation and surgery for individuals with Down's syndrome. Facial transplantation is considered in Chapter 8.

*'Prophylactic' surgery*

A particularly interesting development in recent years has been the availability of risk-reducing or 'prophylactic' procedures (for example, mastectomy) that now offer choices to people with a high risk of developing various diseases, most notably cancer. The psychosocial impact of these procedures that carry with them the possibility of an altered appearance in the absence of a diagnosed condition is still unclear, since results from an emerging body of literature are equivocal. For example, a prospective study by Hatcher et al. (2001) concluded that prophylactic mastectomies may offer psychological benefits without any negative impact upon body image. A retrospective survey (Hopwood et al. 2000) found only minor degrees of body image deterioration, although more than half the participants felt less physically and sexually attractive after risk-reducing mastectomy and a small minority of women reported serious body image concerns and disappointment. Similarly, around 5 per cent of the participants in a study by Payne et al. (2000) expressed regrets about their decision to undergo this same procedure. Although relieved that their risk of breast cancer had been reduced, their regrets focused around body image and sexuality issues, specifically surgical complications, dissatisfaction with cosmetic outcome, scarring and lack of sensation. Furthermore, a long-term follow-up study has suggested that one-third of patients reported poorer body image satisfaction after prophylactic breast surgery (Frost et al. 2000). Clearly this literature is in its infancy and further research is needed as the number of patients contemplating and undergoing risk-reducing surgery increases. Already it is evident that patients considering such surgery warrant specific information regarding the impact of treatment on body image and appropriate support (including counselling) both before and after treatment. Hatcher and Fallowfield (2003) have suggested that a support group would be beneficial since many women report feeling isolated as a result of not knowing anyone else who has undergone this surgery.

*Laser treatment*

Not all interventions provided through the NHS are surgical. Laser treatment used to treat port wine stains was initially hailed as being a 'miracle cure' and patients may have high expectations about the outcome of this prolonged and often painful procedure (Augustin et al. 1998). However, the results of laser treatment can be uneven and it is rare for the blemish to be removed completely. Hansen et al. (2003) conducted an assessment of the longer-term psychological impact of pulse-dyed laser therapy among patients with port wine stains. Sixty-two per cent reported an improvement in colour but few reported any change in texture or size of their port wine stain and most reported that the treatment had not significantly affected their social interactions with other people. In other words, treatment had little impact on psychosocial issues.

### Camouflage services

#### Make-up services

Patients may also be offered prosthetics and camouflage make-up services that essentially aspire to disguise their appearance. These are likely to be adopted by those who are self-conscious about their appearance, in order to lessen its immediate impact, particularly in social situations. It is important to remember that the use of camouflage techniques is by no means unique to people with a visible difference: we all modify or disguise our appearance according to the way in which we appraise a situation and the impression we wish to project.

While clothing can hide disfigurements affecting the limbs and trunk relatively easily, facial disfigurements are usually more difficult to conceal. However, pigment disorders on the face or body (vitiligo or port wine stains) can often be effectively disguised with camouflage make-up (Harris 1997), yet some conditions are difficult to conceal in this way. For example the flaking nature of psoriasis makes this problematic, although not impossible. Unlike cosmetic products, camouflage make-up does not rub off and is waterproof. In the UK, camouflage make-up that can be used on the face and body is available on the NHS via the British Red Cross. Research among patients with port wine stains (Lanigan and Cotterill 1989) has found that women are more likely than men to use camouflage make-up. This may reflect men's reluctance to use products associated with femininity or alternatively, camouflage make-up may be offered to women as a possible intervention strategy more frequently than it is to men. It has also been suggested (Spicer 2002) that camouflage services are not always offered to older people, possibly because of an erroneous belief that the visibility of dermatological conditions is less of a concern for them than it is for younger people.

Regarding the framework offered in Chapter 2, camouflage make-up might successfully cover a disfigurement to a greater or lesser degree which may in turn influence the cognitive representation and feedback an individual receives about their appearance. Since having a variety of coping strategies is thought to be associated with more favourable psychosocial outcomes (see Chapter 5), cosmetic camouflage can be a useful addition to the repertoire of strategies available to an individual and should ideally be offered to all patients as part of standard care.

However, make-up is not a wholly effective remedy and will not necessarily address patients' anxieties about their appearance. This was evident in an evaluation of a skin camouflage service (Kent 2002) that reported high levels of satisfaction with the service, increased confidence in social settings and reduced avoidance, yet participants' core beliefs about appearance and levels of social anxiety remained unchanged. Indeed, the promotion of camouflage make-up services may encourage the belief that a visible difference should be hidden or rectified as opposed to promoting the wider acceptance of a broad range of appearances.

Cosmetic camouflage becomes a problem where it is too heavily relied upon, with people feeling that they cannot face anyone without it. It can bring its own problems in relation to issues of identity and the 'real me', overreliance on the camouflaged image in social interaction, avoidance of 'revealing' situations such as swimming and fears that the 'truth' will be discovered (Coughlan and Clarke 2002). Further problems can be caused if injudicious use draws attention to the disfigurement rather than distracts from it. This is also true of inappropriate clothing, for example continually wearing long-sleeved polo-necked jumpers in order to conceal the arms and neck, even in hot weather. When this happens, camouflage can be seen to have become an avoidance strategy rather than a positive coping strategy.

Individuals relying on camouflage make-up might also find themselves facing an interesting dilemma resulting from the dissonance between the belief that appearance doesn't matter and their behaviour of trying to attain an ideal appearance. While make-up is used in order to aspire to a 'normal' appearance, societal ideals are that appearance should be 'artless'; excessive, obvious use of make-up may be interpreted by some as indicating preoccupation with appearance (see Chapter 2). Clearly this dilemma is not only faced by those with a disfigurement.

*Prosthetics*

Prosthetics can also be considered a form of camouflage. In some instances, for example after mastectomy, patients may elect to use a prosthesis as opposed to undergoing reconstructive surgery. Elsewhere (for example after lower limb amputation) reconstructive surgery is not feasible and prosthetics may be the only option presented (Harris 1997). Prostheses may aim to restore function in addition to normalizing appearance, for example after limb amputation. Much attention has been directed towards the development of improved techniques for the production of more life-like prosthesis, included matching them to a range of skin tones. However, while they can conceal a disfigurement they do not suit everyone and an individual who is adjusting to an altered appearance is also faced with adjusting to the use of a prosthesis. Some women who have used breast prostheses have reported them to be an inconvenient, embarrassing, uncomfortable reminder of the surgery that has taken place and a motivation towards choosing to undergo reconstructive surgery (Reaby and Hort 1995). It is possible that individuals may therefore invest as much attention upon concealing a prosthesis as they did upon disguising their original disfigurement. Yet for others, the prosthesis is an integral part of their identity which they may prefer to display rather than conceal. For example, anecdotal reports of teenagers who choose to sport highly coloured prosthetic devices abound. MacLachlan (2004) describes the notion of embodiment in relation to prostheses, with the prosthesis sometimes becoming incorporated into the body image. Interestingly, he cites the example of a woman who was more distressed when her prosthetic legs were replaced than she was when she originally had her legs amputated following a fire.

In summary, camouflage by way of make-up, clothing or prosthetics is clearly helpful in some circumstances but is not a panacea for all the problems encountered by those who are troubled by their appearance (whether or not they have a visible difference).

## The limitations of a biomedical approach

The surgical and medical interventions just described are provided within a health care system based on the biomedical model. Undoubtedly bio-medical interventions have offered benefits to many patients, in part by modifying the feedback (the reality of physical appearance) that informs self-appraisal. It is important to remember that the successes of advances in treatment are not only the main focus for the NHS, but often for patients themselves. While the belief in the 'fix it' basis of modern health care prevails, biomedical interventions may be the only option available or offered to individuals, who may be unaware that alternatives exist elsewhere. However, these interventions are not a universal remedy and there are a number of limitations with the biomedical approach in this context. While many patients report enhanced self-esteem, more positive appearance ratings, and/or improvements in social confidence following surgery, the results are not clear cut and benefits of surgery cannot be guaranteed (Hughes 1998).

The main problem is that a biomedical approach takes an ostensibly pathological approach by assuming there is a positive relationship between severity and disability (see Clarke 1999). So while it is increasingly recognized that a visible difference could have consequences for the indi-vidual concerned, it is invariably assumed that this will have a negative rather than positive impact and will be greater among those with a more severe or extensive disfigurement. Translating this into the provision of care means that individuals with a more obvious or larger disfigurement are given priority over those whose visible difference is less extensive and by implication deemed less worthy of treatment. However, as previous chapters have shown, research evidence does not necessarily support this assumed and simplistic relationship and has repeatedly demonstrated the importance of psychosocial factors in determining adjustment. Furthermore, the bio-medical model not only presumes a positive relationship between severity of disfigurement and psychosocial distress but also assumes that this is uni–directional. In contrast, a biopsychosocial approach is bi–directional and recognizes that psychological distress could influence the physical characteristics of some conditions (for example, dermatological conditions).

The inadequacy of a solely biomedical approach to care is illustrated particularly well in the provision of services for people with appearance-related conditions where care is typically based upon the surgical and medical interventions outlined earlier. Essentially, the focus is still on interventions to address patients' physical requirements – i.e. 'fixing' appearance with the aim of achieving the perceived norm (an appearance devoid of any obvious difference). The underlying premise is that any biomedical intervention that produces even mild or partial aesthetic improvement is desirable and worthwhile. This serves to promote negative stereotypes and perceptions of any appearance that fails to meet society's exacting standards and reinforces beliefs that individuals with a visible difference should aspire to the norm of a non–disfigured appearance. Meanwhile the increasing availability of surgical interventions for all individuals (whether they have a visible difference or not) fuels prevailing beauty myths and the stereotypes that appearance is important and that what is beautiful is good (see Chapter 1). Cultural ideals to which individuals compare themselves through the cognitive processes outlined in Chapters 2 and 5 are informed and an expectation that individuals should pursue any available treatment or surgery that might 'improve' their appearance is reinforced. This can place further pressure upon individuals who may in effect be putting their life 'on hold' while awaiting a miraculous change and can be especially pertinent if individuals believe that 'fixing' their appearance will also remedy other problems in their lives. There is strong anecdotal evidence of the shock and disappointment experienced when individuals realize that painful, costly, prolonged surgery has not necessarily delivered an ideal life. Partridge (1990) and Bradbury and Middleton (1997) have discussed the importance of recognizing the point at which further treatment incurs more costs than benefits. While a surgeon might continue to aspire to an ideal aesthetic result, many people with a visible disfigurement want to be unremarkable rather than 'perfect' and may need to call a halt to the disruption of surgery and the associated roller coaster of emotions (Bradbury and Middleton 1997; Pruzinsky 2002).

A further problem with biomedical care is that increasingly it is delivered in line with guidelines and protocols that may contradict an individual, person-centred approach. Slavish adherence to rigid surgical protocols in order to 'rectify' appearance (for example, the expectation that cleft-affected patients will undergo jaw surgery in early adolescence) can be unhelpful, exerting undue pressure to undergo a prescribed surgical intervention. This can make it difficult for those affected to participate in decision making and causes considerable disruption to daily life. Rather than imposing inflexible regimes, care needs to be planned to take account of individual physical (for example, growth) and psychosocial issues.

Meanwhile, while an increasing array of options are available to alter physical appearance, less attention is paid to meeting individuals' psychosocial needs or considering the wider context in which treatment and care takes place. This is illustrated by the small amount of funding necessary to maintain an NHS specialist disfigurement support unit (Outlook – see Chapter 7) as opposed to the heavy investment in biomedical interventions, paralleling the widespread priority given to biomedical treatment over psychosocial care for health conditions.

Yet despite the investment in biomedical interventions they cannot be guaranteed to remove body dissatisfaction or restore a patient's appearance to their pre-morbid state. Media messages, together with increasing availability of aesthetic and cosmetic techniques, have encouraged beliefs that surgeons can accomplish far more than is possible. Examples of this include scarring and skin blemishes, with the popular notion that they can be removed. The number of people living with scarring after treatment is significant: it has been suggested that 100 million people in the developed world develop a scar each year (Sund 2000, cited in Bayat et al. 2003), including around 80 million as a result of surgery and 11 million scars are keloid (raised and coloured). The reality is that scarring can often be improved (in the sense of being made less noticeable to an observer) and medical and surgical developments in this area are welcome (Partridge and Rumsey 2003). Developments in laparoscopic surgical techniques have the potential to reduce the need for large incisions and hence reduced scarring, but it is still impossible to remove physical scars completely and psychological scarring (including memories of the possibly traumatic circumstances that led to the scarring) often remains.

Importantly, patients' and health care professionals' understandings of the aims and potential outcomes of any biomedical treatment may not concur. While surgeons and other health care professionals might conceive 'better' to mean that scarring or a blemish is not as extensive or prominent as it had been previously, the patient might equate 'better' as meaning cure or complete removal. Storry (cited in Lansdown et al. 1997) gives a vivid personal illustration of the potential for disappointment when a patient's expectations and understandings of treatment do not match those of their treating physicians:

> Technically the surgeons have done a wonderful job. I can breathe through my nostrils but I am bitterly disappointed at the aesthetic result. I have a bridge but my nose remains flat. I have a problem and I had assumed that the NHS would identify the cause and recommend a series of operations to correct it. I soon learn that my assumption is naïve. If I am to make progress, I will have to cajole the surgeon to undertake further surgery.
>
> (p. 33)

Managing patients' expectations of outcome has become a major challenge for health professionals in this field and health psychologists have a role to play in this respect (see Chapter 7).

A more comprehensive approach recognizes the need to identify psycho-social concerns and to provide appropriate care to address these issues. In addition to improved psychological wellbeing, Dropkin (1999) suggests that there may be direct, medical and economic benefits of helping a patient to adjust to any treatment-induced changes to their appearance, since failure to do so might contribute to reduced adherence to treatment and increased incidence of infections. Similarly, the outcome of many procedures depends on ongoing adherence to treatment regimes. For example a child who has undergone cleft surgery may be required to wear an orthodontic plate after the operation and burn-injured patients may need to wear pressure garments in order to improve the aesthetic outcome of scarring. Adherence to treatment by people without a visible difference might also be influenced by its perceived impact on appearance, for example if a prescribed medication is believed to cause weight gain.

In summary, despite major advances in treatment, it is becoming increasingly evident that care provision based solely on a biomedical model is not sufficient to meet patients' needs in full. Indeed, research with out-patients with a range of visible differences has found that their psycho-social needs were not being met in the clinic context (Rumsey et al. 2004; Rumsey 2003b) and, furthermore, health care staff themselves recognized that these concerns were not being addressed. Reasons given for this mirrored those reported elsewhere in the literature (see Price 1990) and included a lack of time, training, resources, expertise, knowledge, confidence and guidance in how to deal with such issues. The good news is that issues such as expertise and training are amenable to intervention and change and health psychologists have a valuable contribution to make in this context.

## Provision of psychosocial care

It is clear to us, as health psychologists, that the advances and benefits offered by a biomedical approach could be enhanced by incorporating psycho-social care and support into routine health care, in the same way that all patients are offered analgesia, routine physiotherapy and so on. While all health care professionals are in a position to offer psychosocial support during their contact with patients, pressures on staff and workloads may mean that psychosocial care and support is not always available when needed. In this section we first consider the benefits offered by a biopsycho-social approach and then examine the current provision of psychosocial care for people with visible differences.

Readers are directed towards Engel (1977) and Ogden (2004) for an overview of a biopsychosocial approach and its perceived advantages over the biomedical model. With specific reference to appearance research and practice, a biopsychosocial is preferable since it does not focus solely on 'fixing' appearance. Rather it takes a broader view and reflects the social nature of the problems typically encountered by those with a visible difference. It recognizes that helping individuals to change their thoughts, feelings and behaviours in relation to their looks is as relevant (or more so) than changing their objective physical appearance. As mentioned previously, it is also bi-directional in recognizing that psychosocial factors can influence the physical aspects of disease and vice versa. However, it is not without its limitations and has been criticized for not being sufficiently distinct from a biomedical approach and for being unable to meet the high expectations made of it (see Marks et al. (2000) for an overview).

While the overarching conceptual framework of 'disfigurement' *per se* (see Chapter 2) is useful, clinical services are typically focused and organized around specific conditions. A useful way of evaluating the provision of care is to consider whether appearance-related concerns are acknowledged and/or addressed.

Where the condition has been more intensively investigated from a psychological perspective, there are likely to be more services in place. Thus, there is a long-standing body of evidence pointing to the importance of psychosocial factors in cleft, burn care and breast cancer. Most burns units, cleft and breast cancer teams now have well-established protocols to provide psychosocial care in the short term, although long-term care tends to be less well established. The recognition of psychosocial issues is clearly evident in policy relating to provision of care for these conditions. For example, following work by the Clinical Standards Advisory Group (CSAG 1998) a government circular recommended the inclusion of 'an appropriately trained psychologist' in each new cleft team in the UK. Within cancer care, the NHS Cancer Plan (2000) and the Calman–Hine Report (1995) have stressed the need for patients' psychosocial needs to be addressed at every stage of their care. This has often been provided by specialist nurses with training in counselling skills. The National Burns Care Committee (2001) has outlined the importance of psychosocial support and suggested the basis for a UK national standard. However, these policy recommendations and guidelines may not be translated into improved services and care unless there is sufficient funding and incentive. In reality a patient may not receive such idealized support: a survey of psychological need among 71 burn-injured patients (Kleve and Robinson 1999) found that only 39 per cent reported having received support for the emotional effects of the injury while they were inpatients. Since these tended to be the patients who were admitted for a longer period of time, there may have been more time to provide them with psychological support. Alternatively, since care was provided within a biomedical setting, assumptions about a link between severity and distress may have resulted in only those with more extensive burns being offered support. While 66 per cent of respondents reported receiving support after leaving hospital (from their GP, family) only 4 per cent had had contact with a psychologist or psychiatrist after discharge. Again, this finding can be interpreted in numerous ways: while it might indicate that other members of the care team had developed skills enabling them to provide the necessary support, it could also reflect an unmet need. Indeed at the time of the survey, 38 per cent felt they would benefit from some kind of professional help.

It is clear that some conditions are not only recognized as having an impact upon appearance but also that concerns are expected and are invariably deemed to have a negative impact. In these situations psychological distress as a result of an altered appearance is often seen as the norm, particularly for those with extensive disfiguration and, furthermore, psychosocial care and support may be provided. The irony of this raised awareness is the danger that psychosocial needs of those with mild or moderate disfigurement will be overlooked in the erroneous assumption that they will be less distressed (see Chapter 4).

In contrast, other conditions may have no specialist psychological services at all, possibly because of a lack of research evidence to verify its need, the relative rarity of the condition or a failure to recognize that the condition might have an impact upon appearance-related distress. For example rheumatoid arthritis and diabetes have an impact upon appearance that may be neither expected by the patient nor addressed by available care. Rather, the functional and physiological aspects of the condition are prioritized and in some cases may be the sole focus of care. However, there is some evidence that a shift is taking place with organizations, such as those supporting people with arthritis, developing support programmes around body image.

Ideally, psychosocial needs in relation to appearance will be acknowledged, identified and addressed through a variety of sources throughout the patient's care. Clearly many clinicians and care teams are aware of the problems their patients encounter on a daily basis. However, many others may be unaware of the extent of appearance-related concerns among the people they care for. It has been suggested (Hopwood and Maguire 1988) that levels of appearance-related concerns may be underestimated since the medical system and health professionals may eschew such issues, thus preventing patients from reporting their concerns for fear of appearing ungrateful, vain or wasting professionals' time. Similarly, health care professionals who are regularly working with patients with an altered appearance may become desensitized to its possible impact for the individual. Vamos (1990) identifies this as a particular issue among those working with people with rheumatoid arthritis. In such circumstances it is unlikely that an individual requiring additional psychosocial support would be identified and referred on. Even where good support is available, the patient's access to such services may be limited, either consciously or unconsciously via gatekeepers.

The variability in individual experiences and responses to appearance may be one reason for the apparent difficulties in meeting patients' psychosocial needs adequately; the variability certainly presents a challenge in terms of designing appropriate screening protocols and strategies for support. While people in Rumsey et al.'s (2004) audit of outpatient attendees were generally happy with the quality of care provided in the clinic, psychological outcomes were positively related to level of involvement in decision making, ease of understanding and provision of information. Clinic staff were generally aware of the difficulties that patients were facing and felt that they could be the most appropriate people to help address those problems but often also felt that they had not been trained to deliver the kind of specialist help needed. There were also some interesting mismatches in care provision. For example in an eye clinic, counselling was routinely offered for patients who were going to lose an eye, whereas the study demonstrated higher levels of distress among patients with thyroid eye disease for whom there was no provision of psychosocial support (see Clarke et al. 2003).

A challenge facing any health care team is to develop an ethos in which appearance concerns can be discussed at every stage of the patient's care and in which people do not feel stigmatized if they are identified as needing psychological support. Pruzinsky (2004) has called for psychological and body image assessment to be incorporated as part of the routine care for any medical condition or disorder. This would be a welcome step towards raising the profile of appearance concerns among people undergoing medical care, but being aware of concerns is one issue; being able to provide appropriate care is another and, as stressed previously, health care professionals may feel unable to meet patients' needs. For example, a survey of specialist head and neck cancer nurses (Clarke and Cooper 2001) found that respondents did not feel sufficiently skilled in offering this care. It is likely that staff working in other specialties would also report greater confidence in providing physical as opposed to psychosocial care.

People with appearance-related concerns (including those with a visible difference) might find themselves referred to non-specialist services (including health and clinical psychologists) without any particular expertise in appearance and disfigurement issues. In addition to the problem of limited experience, such a system will tend to be reactive as opposed to proactive and while these services may offer a range of useful general support services, clear referral routes to psychologists with expertise in appearance are needed. Unfortunately such services are few and far between so that access and availability to such services is difficult at best. However, the specialist services that do exist offer a useful model for future care provision (details in Chapter 7).

**Legal intervention**

On a wider scale, UK law offers a stick that could impact positively upon the experiences and quality of life of people with a visible difference. As a result of campaigning by support organizations for those affected, the Disability Discrimination Act (1995) now specifically includes 'severe disfigurement' as a disability. Benefits of the Act are that it specifically gives rights in the areas of employment, access to services, goods, facilities (including health care), buying and renting land and property. With regard to disfigurement, the Act does not require the individual to demonstrate that the disfigurement has a substantial adverse effect on their ability to carry out normal day-to-day activities (the definition of physical disability employed by the Act). Yet while it is now an offence to discriminate against anyone on the basis of their appearance, enforcement of such a law is plagued with difficulty since evidence will be hard to collate and prove. For example, who is to dictate whether or not an individual's disfigurement is 'severe' and how would this be achieved? Furthermore, it could be difficult to provide evidence that an individual was discriminated against, for example at a job interview, on the basis of their appearance. The impact of this legislation upon the lives of people with a visible difference remains to be seen.

**Conclusion**

In summary, current health service provision for appearance-related concerns is based principally on the biomedical model, with variable and generally sparse provision of psychosocial services. We applaud the developments in biomedical interventions and cannot, nor would we want to, change this. Rather, there is a need to ensure psychosocial issues are given a place alongside or ahead of medical and surgical treatments. In some instances, appearance issues are recognized and provided for, as evidenced by the availability of plastic and reconstructive surgery, while in other areas they are given scant attention. Although psychological support is routinely available and sometimes seen as a priority in areas such as eating disorders, body dysmorphia and (increasingly) prophylactic surgery, on the whole the provision of appropriate care and support for most individuals falls short of an ideal. This presents interesting challenges for psychologists working in this area. Clearly, changing the ethos of care in relation to appearance issues is an uphill struggle when the biomedical model is so established and entrenched in training and practice. It has been encouraging to see how research evidence has led to a growing emphasis on the importance of psychological input in guidelines for the provision of care among a range of conditions, for example within burns care. Yet most psychosocial care is still reactive rather than proactive and most support is provided through the voluntary sector, putting increasing pressure on them to raise funds to cover their costs.

Regarding care and support for individuals without a visible difference, the options beyond self-management are currently limited. There is a notable dearth of research into interventions that might prevent the development of appearance dissatisfaction (Liossi 2003). The potential for more effective support and intervention is very promising and the following chapter considers examples of ways in which psychosocial care and issues might be addressed.

## Chapter summary

♦ Attempts to address appearance-related concerns and dissatisfaction involve altering either an individual's objective physical appearance or the cognitive processes by which their appearance is appraised and evaluated;

♦ In the majority of instances, individuals attempting to change their appearance do so without professional or surgical intervention, yet an increasing minority elects to undergo privately funded cosmetic surgical and non-surgical interventions;

♦ There is a general dearth of services offering psychological support for individuals with appearance-related concerns, except for those with eating disorders, body dysmorphic disorder or an appearance that is clearly different from 'the norm';

♦ Much of the support available for people who are troubled by a visible difference is provided through the voluntary sector. While support groups will not suit all individuals they can be an invaluable resource for many;

♦ Advances in medical, surgical and cosmetic interventions can be greatly beneficial to many people but it is becoming increasingly evident that care provision that is based solely within a biomedical framework may not be a panacea for all the difficulties encountered by individuals who are visibly different;

♦ Unfortunately the current provision of appropriate care and support for most individuals falls short of an ideal and the potential for more effective support and intervention is great.

## Discussion points

♦ Think about your own experiences as a user of health care services. Were issues of appearance ever relevant and if so, were they addressed? How?

♦ How well do biomedical interventions address appearance-related concerns?

◆ From a psychological perspective, should cosmetic surgery be made freely available to everyone?

## Further reading

Lansdown, R., Rumsey, N., Bradbury, E., Carr, T. and Partridge, J. (eds) (1997) *Visibly Different: Coping with Disfigurement.* Oxford: Butterworth-Heinemann.

Pruzinsky, T. (2004) Enhancing quality of life in medical populations: a vision for body image assessment and rehabilitation as standards of care. *Body Image,* 1: 71–81.

Sarwer, D.B. and Crerand, C.E. (2004) Body image and cosmetic medical treatments. *Body Image,* 1: 99–111.

# The potential for more effective support and intervention

*(with contributions from Alex Clarke)*

Having examined current psychosocial support and interventions for people with appearance-related concerns in the UK (Chapter 6), it is clear that there is much room for improvement. This chapter focuses on possible ways of providing effective, accessible psychosocial care through health care systems and also considers the potential role for educational interventions, the media and health promotion campaigns. The opportunities for health psychologists working in clinical and research settings are many and varied. As before, interventions could be directed towards changing either an individual's objective physical appearance or their attitudes towards it. Comprehensive care should also address individuals' dealings with others and the attitudes they hold. While presented here in a particular order, ideally these interventions would be available simultaneously and accessible for any particular individual, as necessary.

## Interventions directed at the population as a whole

Changing attitudes towards appearance within the population as a whole is a monumental task, but given that 'body dissatisfaction is the common experience of most people raised in Western culture' (Grogan 1999: 189), the potential for change is enormous.

### The media

The influence of the media on the development and reinforcement of appearance-related concerns was discussed in Chapter 3. Clearly it can be a powerful modelling influence for many people. Invariably, reference to the media in this context is couched in negative terms yet there is scope for it to be used to dispel prevailing beauty myths and to encourage a more positive agenda towards appearance within the population as a whole. The advertising industry and television are good illustrations of the influence of the media.

For years, men and women with idealized and unattainable images have enticed us to buy products ranging from air fresheners to zip fasteners. Experimental research has demonstrated that even brief exposure to such images can increase body-focused anxiety (Halliwell and Dittmar 2004) but Halliwell and Dittmar's research found that using 'average' as opposed to 'skinny' models could help to reduce this anxiety. Advertisers' reactions to this research are yet to be gauged. In recent years some successful advertising campaigns (for example for Dove moisturiser in the UK) have featured 'normal' sized models but these remain the exception and tellingly, even when bigger models are used they are still expected to be 'attractive'! Clearly there is some way to go before attainable images are the norm within the media. Ideally, the power of the fashion and beauty industries would be harnessed not only to display more representative images but also to promote positive health behaviours, for example to improve attitudes towards skin protection in the sun (Carmel et al. 1994). However, Naomi Wolf (cited in Grogan 1999) claims this is overoptimistic since the beauty industry has a vested interest in women's dissatisfaction with their appearance.

It is interesting to note that while the advertising of some health-damaging products (for example tobacco) has been banned in the UK, there is currently no legislation to control or restrict advertisements for cosmetic surgery despite the potential risks associated with it. Rather, they are more prominent and widespread than ever and Grogan (1999) was unable to identify any British magazine aimed at young women that did not include these adverts. Furthermore, they are now just as evident in the growing market of publications aimed at men and are also promoted in television commercials and on poster campaigns in public spaces. The exact extent to which these adverts encourage individuals' dissatisfaction with their appearance remains unclear.

Recent television programmes aired in the UK (for example, *You Are What You Eat* (Channel 4) and *The Big Challenge* (BBC 1)) have aimed to encourage individuals to adopt a healthier lifestyle through diet and exercise. Clearly the participants in these programmes are motivated as much by their desire to change their appearance as they are to improve their health, illustrating how health behaviours are often influenced by factors relating to appearance rather than by health beliefs (Leary et al. 1994). These programmes might go some way towards influencing the perceived social norms regarding a healthy lifestyle. Since research has repeatedly found that people who exercise have higher levels of body image satisfaction and self-esteem than those who do not exercise (see Grogan (1999) for an overview), interventions that promote exercise are a natural follow-on. However, the longer-term effectiveness of media-informed interventions is unclear.

Media images directed towards adolescents could be especially influential given this group's apparent preoccupation with appearance (see Chapter 3). We were recently struck by the powerful impression that an exhibition of paintings by the artist Mark Gilbert (in 1997) had on a group of 16 and 17 year olds. They reported how his portraits of surgical patients (many of whom had head and neck cancer) were strong incentives not to smoke. Haste's (2004) survey of young people (see Chapter 2) found that girls in particular use magazines as a source of information about health issues. Ideally magazines would present alternative views of the importance of appearance to this potentially impressionable age group.

Media campaigns directed towards the population as a whole could also be used to inform attitudes and to promote the acceptance of a greater diversity of appearance. A poster campaign by the charity Changing Faces recently depicted people with a range of facial disfigurements and encouraged observers to engage with them in everyday social interactions with messages including 'If you can hold my gaze we could hold a conversation' (see also Figure 7.1). This award-winning campaign was notable for two reasons. First, it consisted of positive images of people with facial disfigurements, and second, it suggested strategies for how people who are unused to meeting others with a visible difference should act in such circumstances. It seems this advice is needed – a YouGov (2003) opinion poll commissioned by Changing Faces found that 79 per cent of respondents would be scared of doing the wrong thing if they met someone with a severe facial disfigurement.

In 2004 a UK television programme entitled *Celebrities Disfigured* aimed to portray life with a visible difference from the perspectives of a well-known actor and model who were made up to look as if they had burns scarring or a port wine stain. This was a twist on early psychosocial research into the proxemic behaviour of the general public towards individuals with a visible difference (see Chapters 2 and 4). It could be argued that documentaries about the real-life experiences of individuals with genuine disfigurements (such as *The Boy Whose Skin Fell Off* (Channel 4 2004) about one man's life with Epidermolysis Bullosa and *One Life: In Your Face* (BBC 2003) which followed a woman's decision to no longer conceal her facial birthmark) might be preferable and have greater validity. However, a celebrity association is likely to have increased viewing figures and thereby spread the programme's message to a larger audience. Hopefully sensitive and informative programmes help to change attitudes towards appearance and thereby contribute towards improving quality of life for people with a visible difference.

### Health promotion campaigns

The use of the media within health promotion campaigns has been considered at length by Bennett and Murphy (1997). However, few health promotion campaigns have focused explicitly on appearance, despite growing realization that many people engage in health behaviours because

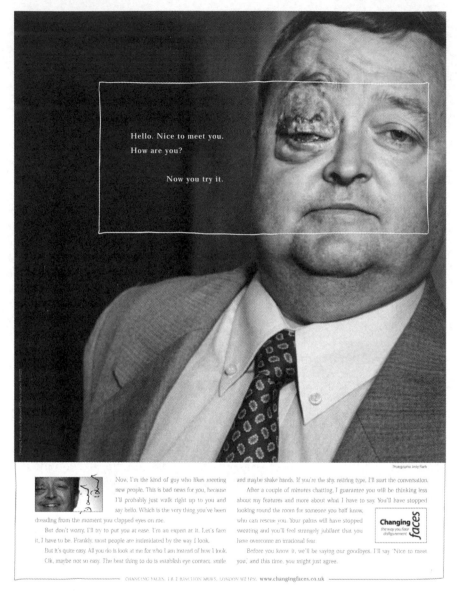

*Figure 7.1*    An example of the Changing Faces poster campaign

of their anticipated impact upon appearance rather than purported health benefits (see Leary et al. (1994) and Chapter 2). Leary et al. (1994: 467) suggested that 'the big question is how to persuade people to pay more attention to their health and less to their public image?' However, given the high importance placed on appearance in current western society it seems more sensible to exploit this interest in appearance as a motivation to change health behaviours positively.

One area in which appearance has driven health promotion campaigns is sun tanning behaviour and skin cancer. A leaflet-based intervention as part of the UK Health Education Authority's 'If You Worship the Sun, Don't Sacrifice Your Skin' campaign (Castle et al. 1999) found that the perceived benefits of having a sun tan (including positive attitude towards physical appearance) predicted intention to suntan without protection. Increasing knowledge about the risks of sun exposure might change risk behaviour, but attitudes towards suntans are, like those towards many health behaviours, deeply entrenched: a study by the American Academy of Dermatology reported that 72 per cent of respondents thought that a suntan looked healthy. Increased knowledge (for example about cancer risk) is unlikely to change behaviour on its own – attitudes also need to be manipulated. Jones and Leary (1994) suggested this could be achieved by promoting images of wrinkles and ageing. Indeed a recent anti-smoking campaign aimed at young women utilized the negative impact that smoking has upon appearance. This was particularly pertinent given the worrying increase in the numbers of smokers in this group for whom we know appearance is a particular concern. Similarly, health warnings on tobacco products in the UK include the statement 'smoking causes aging of the skin' and an array of graphic images soon to be introduced across Europe includes this same warning alongside a photograph of an apple with wrinkled skin.

The difficulty is that the impact of behaviour changes on appearance is not immediate. Wrinkles and ageing, for example, are a problem for the future, whereas perceived benefits such as a suntan, weight control and image are attainable in the shorter term. Some people are more open than others to health promotion campaigns (Bennett and Murphy 1997) and in this instance it is likely to be the salience of appearance that determines receptiveness. For example anti–smoking messages that focus on appearance issues are more likely to be heeded by people who want to avoid premature wrinkles than by those who fear gaining weight if they were to give up. This needs further investigation.

Finally, it is possible that health promotion campaigns that play on appearance concerns may actually reinforce prevailing negative stereotypes such as those surrounding ageing and appearance. This contradicts attempts to promote greater acceptance of diversity of appearance and to dispel the myth that only youthful looks are desirable.

### School-based interventions

Schools offer both an educational and social environment in which to challenge attitudes and myths about the importance of appearance. They could be especially useful since appearance is often a trigger for bullying in schools (Crozier and Dimmock 1999). They also offer an opportunity to support students with a visible difference while enabling other students and staff (including teachers, kitchen staff, caretakers etc.) to mix and interact with those with visible differences. Hopefully this might encourage a greater appreciation of diversity of appearance.

Despite the prevalence of appearance concerns among children and adolescents, there are very few interventions aimed at tackling appearance-related issues among young people who do not have a visible difference. An exception to this has been a classroom-based intervention that was devised and evaluated using an action research methodology (Lovegrove and Rumsey 2005; see also Box 7.1).

---

### Box 7.1  An example of a school-based intervention

Lovegrove and Rumsey (2005) reported an intervention based on those formulated by Changing Faces for use among children with a visible difference. It aimed to educate secondary school pupils about the causes of visible difference, challenge appearance-related myths and generate strategies to tackle their own social difficulties. These strategies included:

◆ devising and practising a positive self-motto;
◆ preparing an explanation for their perceived difference that would reassure other people ('I've got acne, you can't catch it');
◆ taking charge of a conversation by responding neutrally to any negative or bullying comments;
◆ making use of friends.

Results showed significant improvements in body image, self-esteem and social confidence relative to non-intervention controls, with improvements maintained at six-month follow-up. One of the benefits of this approach is the ease with which materials can be used by trained teaching staff, so that specialist psychological input would not be necessary at every session.

---

However, such pro-active interventions are only likely to be taken up by schools and staff with an awareness of the magnitude and impact of appearance-related concerns among adolescent groups. A coordinated programme is needed to raise awareness of the problems, offer possible interventions and evaluate such activity among school populations.

### Support within health care systems

Chapter 6 highlighted the relative dearth of psychosocial support for appearance issues within any health care system. Ideally, support relating to appearance should be part of routine health care for all conditions and treatments (Pruzinsky 2002). This requires all health care staff to have an awareness of the possible negative psychosocial impact of appearance concerns. Many issues experienced by those with appearance concerns (particularly problems such as poor sexual functioning) will not be picked up at all unless there are clear protocols for psychological assessment (via clinical interviews or use of assessment measures) in routine care. The difficulty lies in maintaining a balance between creating an ethos of care in which appearance issues are an important and pertinent focus without setting expectations that such concerns are inevitable. Health psychologists have a role to play in raising awareness among health care professionals, training staff to identify individuals who may benefit from further support and designing, delivering and evaluating appropriate interventions.

Liossi (2003) discussed the potential benefit of appearance dissatisfaction treatment programmes among individuals without a visible difference. She suggests they should be based on the principles of cognitive behavioural therapy, similar to the structure of Cash's approach (see Chapter 6) and should target appearance schemacity, negative thoughts about body image, cognitive errors in evaluating appearance, dysfunctional behavioural strategies and psychological distress about appearance. Liossi also suggests that individuals should be encouraged to develop strategies to develop a more positive attitude towards their appearance (for example, by taking up a sport). This would have associated physical health benefits as well as reducing body dissatisfaction.

## Improving support for people with a visible difference

The suggestions and aspirations outlined earlier could prove beneficial to everyone with concerns about their appearance, regardless of whether or not they have a visible difference. In addition, it is imperative that the particular, individual needs of those with a visible difference are given close attention so that those who might benefit from psychosocial intervention are identified and appropriate support can be made available.

In Chapter 6 we stressed that even the most successful surgical interventions are unlikely to remove all traces of a visible difference. An individual is still likely to have an appearance that is somewhat different to 'the norm' and interventions and care that address their psychosocial needs are vital. The benefits of psychosocial as opposed to surgical interventions were neatly summed up by Cochrane and Slade (1999: 499) when they stated that 'facilitating positive appraisals and adaptive coping may be as, or more, important than the objective aesthetics of surgical outcomes'.

We now consider two ways in which psychosocial care and support should be made available and delivered. First, as general psychological support for all patients as part of routine care (including the acute phase of treatment or primary care) and second, as specific problem-focused interventions designed and delivered by psychologists or trained health care professionals.

While the focus here is on the role played by health care and voluntary support organizations, it is important not to overlook the contribution made by family and friends whose support may be more constant and readily available than that provided by any one professional or organization. (The importance of social support as a factor in determining adjustment was examined in Chapter 5.) Indeed, a study of orofacial cancer patients' ratings of sources of support (Broomfield et al. 1997) confirmed the importance of family and friends while problems were identified with the support received from the primary care sector, community nurses and other patients.

### General psychological support

The opportunity to integrate psychosocial care into routine care delivered by appropriately trained health care professionals has been illustrated by Dropkin (1989) and is simply accomplished, for example in discussion of coping strategies for managing altered appearance while engaged in other care activities such as attending to dressings. This makes this model of care one of the most readily achieved and practical to deliver. It may also facilitate an ethos of care in which appearance issues are a recognized and credible concern within which patients feel more able to discuss such issues.

A comprehensive system of psychosocial care includes providing any necessary support during decision making about treatment, ensuring patients have appropriate information to meet their individual needs and identifying those in need of specialist support.

### Identifying those in need of specialist support

Routine assessment for concerns about appearance is one way of identifying those who might benefit from specialist support. Ideally, every care team and consultant working in an appearance-related specialty would have a designated psychologist working with them and seeing every patient at clinic attendance. However, since resources are typically limited, screening by a psychologist can be targeted and focused upon times of known difficulties. For example, research within cleft care has shown that 7/8 years of age is a time at which most teasing takes place, while transfer to a new school around 10 years of age is also a particularly stressful time for many young people. Specialist psychological input might be especially valuable at these times, but other health care staff have an invaluable role to play beyond these times. This can involve them sensitively ascertaining whether patients are avoiding activities because of their appearance (for example not looking at themselves in mirrors, avoiding social situations) and referring on any patients who are identified as warranting support. Unfortunately recent research (Clarke and Cooper 2001; Clarke et al. 2003; Rumsey et al. 2004) has shown a lack of clear processes to identify those patients who might benefit from support and identified a need to raise the profile of psychosocial issues in this setting.

One problem is that staff may find the prospect of screening patients a formidable task. It is easy to understand why clinicians are enthusiastic towards standardized measures with predetermined cut-off scores to identify those patients deemed to warrant further support. However, while a 'scores on the doors' approach such as this would be relatively quick and cheap, it is unlikely to detect individuals' specific appearance-related concerns. Clarke offers examples of questions as an alternative (see Box 7.2) means of identifying patients' appearance-related concerns. These were developed by the organization Changing Faces and intended to help health care staff raise psychosocial issues with their patients.

Once those who may benefit from psychosocial support have been identified it is imperative for there to be protocols for referral routes to specialist services (such as those detailed below) in order for them to have speedy access to appropriate care.

### Supporting patient decision making

While many patients (or in the case of children, their parents) may be faced with a bewildering array and succession of decisions about their treatment (Chapter 6), others may not feel they have been involved in decisions about interventions that may have an obvious and sometimes permanent impact upon their physical appearance. This can be an especially pertinent issue for more 'vulnerable' groups such as older people or adolescents. Turner et al. (1997) reported that 23 per cent of 15 year olds in a sample of patients with clefts felt excluded from treatment decisions, which presumably had been made by their parents and health care professionals.

Not all patients appreciate the responsibility of decision making and prefer to leave 'the experts' to 'problem-solving' tasks (such as identifying a 'correct solution' to a medical problem) requiring specialist knowledge (Deber et al. 1996). Rather, they may want to participate when choices with different risks and trade-offs are available and when patient preference is a viable option. Decisions relating to appearance often fit these criteria. For example choosing to undergo further surgery to 'improve' appearance involves weighing up perceived costs and benefits. Selecting a particular procedure may have implications for scarring and the anticipated cosmetic results of alternative techniques may vary while decisions regarding a series of reconstructive operations could involve choices about the timing of each procedure. Comprehensive care involves establishing the extent to which patients wish to be involved, facilitating this process for them and realizing that their desire for involvement may change over time and according to the decision being made.

---

**Box 7.2    A simple psychological screening process for identifying patients' appearance-related concerns**

*Step One*
   How do you think that the change in your appearance will affect your life, if at all?

*If patient indicates no impact, confirm with a statement:*
   So there is nothing that you think you will feel uncomfortable about when you first go home?
   If yes, go on to Step Two, if no, go on to Step Three.

*Step Two*
   What are the specific things that you feel less comfortable about?
   (*list three examples*)

*Step Three*
   Sometimes patients ask what to do when other people ask questions about their (use patient's condition as the example). I'd be interested to hear what kind of thing you think that you might do.
   (*record response*)

*Step Four – Observations of behaviour during the assessment*
   Did the patient avoid making eye contact with you? Y/N
   Did the patient try to conceal their face by turning to one side or covering their face with their hand? Y/N

*Step Five – Action planning*
   Based on the patient's verbal and non-verbal responses to your questions, do you think there are any social or emotional consequences of the change in their appearance?

Yes/No/Maybe (*circle one*)

If your answer is 'yes' or 'maybe' will you:

♦ Suggest that they speak to the psychologist?
♦ Ask the psychologist to speak to them?
♦ Offer them relevant information?
♦ Suggest a coping strategy yourself?

---

Support should be available to facilitate patients' decision making, particularly for those finding this difficult. Interviews with 103 women who had been offered breast reconstruction (Harcourt and Rumsey 2004) found that a small subset found this decision particularly difficult for two reasons. First, they could not identify an aspect of mastectomy or reconstruction that was especially salient to them as an individual. This contrasted with those who found decision making relatively easy. For example, some women felt it was personally salient not to use a prosthesis and this was sufficient to facilitate a relatively easy-to-make decision in favour of reconstructive surgery. Second, those who found decision making particularly difficult reported that information and advice offered by other people, including health care professionals increased rather than alleviated their confusion and uncertainty. For example:

> . . . I can trust his judgement so it didn't take me long to decide to do what he said. Then the breast care nurse said 'well, if you're not sure why don't you just have the mastectomy with a prosthesis and then have the reconstruction later?' Well, I've got to be honest with you, but that really mixed me up. I hadn't even thought about that, so my head was spinning again. It's stupid, I didn't know what to think of that . . .
>
> (Harcourt and Rumsey 2004: 112)

Sensitive and emotive decisions such as those relating to appearance are not made in line with theories of decision making that assume rationality. This is partly because they are not made in a social vacuum and attention needs to be given to the role and influence of health care professionals and significant others on individuals' appearance-related decision making. For example in the study outlined above, health care professionals' use of the words 'disfigured' and 'deformed' created a negative image of mastectomy that influenced women's decisions to elect reconstructive surgery (Harcourt and Rumsey 2004). Clarifying patient priorities, attitudes, knowledge and confidence in decision making can be useful and may make it easier to provide appropriate information.

### Information and self-help materials

Provision of clear, relevant information is an example of how helpful interventions need not be costly or time consuming and can be made available to all. This is particularly useful since, given the number of people with concerns about their appearance, it would be a formidable task to even attempt to offer them all psychosocial support through specific interventions such as those outlined here (Newell 2000a). Furthermore, such interventions might not suit all individuals or meet their specific needs.

The best model of care is where information can be provided in response to a clearly identified need and then reviewed with a patient and further questions or explanations dealt with. One way of doing this is to clearly establish the patient's information needs and concerns at any particular time. Various attempts have been made to develop and implement interventions that might facilitate this process. For example, Ambler et al. (1999) reported an intervention that encouraged patients to prepare for their consultation by eliciting a list of questions they wanted addressed and enabled a specialist nurse to act as their advocate in the consultation, if necessary. While this particular intervention was evaluated among patients awaiting the outcome of tests that might lead to a diagnosis of cancer, this approach may prove beneficial in many other situations; for example preparing for discussions about possible plastic or reconstructive surgery.

Written information in conjunction with face-to-face discussions can be very helpful in establishing an appropriate and preferred vocabulary with which to describe appearance and facilitate discussions about appearance at any stage. For example, Clarke and Kish (1998) developed a booklet for use by parents with their children, to give them a shared vocabulary with which to develop appropriate coping strategies for use in social situations, and especially at school.

Clarke (2001) described an information series that uses social cognition and coping models to help individuals understand their problems in a social context, modify any negative beliefs and encourage the use of a range of coping strategies with the aim of facilitating active participation in the management of their condition. Patients' needs for information are endorsed by the number of requests made to organizations such as Changing Faces and by the popularity of NHS Direct. Such requests can be seen partly as attempts by the individual to be proactive and to take control of the management of their situation. Leaflets are clearly popular with patients and leaflet-based interventions can be both cost-effective and beneficial to patients. Newell and Clarke (2000) evaluated the use of a self-help leaflet containing explanations of the relationships between anxiety, changes to facial appearance and avoidance and described a range of practical cognitive-behavioural strategies to address appearance-related anxiety. The intervention, based on Newell's fear-avoidance model (see Chapter 2), resulted in modest but significant improvements in both social and general anxiety. Spicer (2002) found that almost a quarter of participants in her study of people over the age of 65 attending an outpatient dermatology clinic would welcome appearance-related information in leaflet form.

There are both advantages and disadvantages to the ease with which written information can be provided. One particular difficulty in this area is that the aesthetic outcome of surgical intervention cannot be predicted for any particular individual, even if the likelihood of possible side effects and complications is known. There is a danger of disappointment if a patient unrealistically expects that the results of their surgery will match the images contained in mass-produced self-help materials. Patients have expressed a desire for a wider range of post-operative images to be made available, to include individuals with a range of physiques, ages and skin colour (Harcourt and Rumsey 2004). Furthermore, information that focuses on post-operative appearance may leave patients unprepared in other ways, for example the impact in terms of altered sensation, body image and possible discomfort.

Audio and videotapes can be useful sources of information for patients and provide, as with written information, the opportunity for relatives and carers to be involved. A ward or outpatient library offering this kind of information or access to a computer with quality-controlled information via recommended websites provides an exciting opportunity to integrate information from the best different sources. While there may be concerns that such information may not be evidence-based, websites offered by responsible informed organizations can be a valuable resource. Research among other disease groups including those affected by HIV illnesses and diabetes has shown the Internet to be an effective resource for people with chronic conditions (see Bennett 2004) and there is no reason to believe that it could not offer similar benefits to individuals with appearance concerns. Although requiring a degree of expert support in the development and maintenance of such interventions (Bennett 2004), the Internet offers the potential for specialized information to be readily available to all those affected; not only those who are in a geographical location that gives them easy access to specialist services.

Advances in other aspects of computer technology also have the potential to offer innovative means of information provision and support. For example, morphing software is being employed by surgeons to explore potential changes to appearance through surgical interventions. McGarvey et al. (2001) described the use of computer imaging to enable women to prepare themselves in advance of possible chemotherapy-induced hair loss. Supported by a psychologist, patients viewed a simulation of their hair loss before treatment began in the belief that the opportunity to see this image and to express the emotions that it generates would enable the patient to anticipate and deal more easily with any real hair loss. However, the authors gave anecdotal rather than research evidence for the benefits of this intervention and individual differences dictate that this type of intervention will not suit all patients, since information needs and coping strategies vary. Indeed it is possible that it may heighten appearance anxieties unnecessarily and in extreme cases could lead patients to decline treatment. In addition, this particular type of intervention would require considerable resources and have staffing implications. Furthermore, patients who have experienced chemotherapy-induced alopecia report that no amount of warning about possible hair loss could prepare them for the full impact of the actual loss (Williams et al. 1999).

*Support in the post-treatment period*

Seeing the results of treatment or an altered appearance for the first time is a significant and possibly shocking time for many patients. A survey of 222 nurses caring for burn-injured patients (Birdsall and Weinberg 2001) found that the patient's first sight of a wound was usually an unrecorded, unplanned event. Respondents thought that patients often saw their changed looks for the first time in mirrored or reflective surfaces, which may indicate their desire to see their altered appearance as soon as possible but also suggests that they may be unprepared. While this study examined nurses' perceptions as opposed to the patient's own experience, personal accounts (Partridge 1990) concur with their findings that this is a major yet often unplanned event. Kwasi Afari-Mintu survived the King's Cross fire on the London underground in 1987. In a vivid and moving account of his experiences since the fire he describes how he first saw the burns on his face:

> . . . I managed to get to the loo on my own . . . and was washing my hands when I just happened to look into the mirror and I saw this strange person looking back. I couldn't believe it. I stood there for a while, just rooted to the spot. I just couldn't believe it. In fact, I ran my hand over my face to make sure that I was the person I was looking at, and then I felt very, very sorry for myself. I realized I'd been changed into something else. I hung on to the sink for twenty or thirty minutes and just cried. It was the first time I really cried.
>
> (in Lansdown et al. 1997: 56)

Protocols in this respect vary. Care for people with burn injuries leads the way, with standards of care stressing this must be handled with particular care, patients must be prepared, careful consideration must be given to the appropriate timing and support must be on hand (National Burns Care Committee 2001). Further research needs to examine practice in a range of specialties (for example, general plastics, amputation) in order to enable recommendations for good practice elsewhere. In addition to seeing the reality of their own altered appearance, the individual also has to deal with the reactions of other people when they first see their altered looks. These significant others may also benefit from psychosocial care at this stage and appropriate support can facilitate communication between family members at this difficult time (Bradbury 1997).

Returning home after surgery or trauma may not be an exclusively positive event since the hospital environment can offer a degree of security and protection from the stress of 'the real world' where the individual might encounter negative reactions towards their looks for the first time. This could be especially pertinent for those who have had a prolonged period of hospitalization (after serious burns for example) and who have become accustomed to being among other people with a similar appearance but will now be visibly distinctive from those around them. Partridge (1990) vividly describes his experiences in this respect. Appropriate support and infor-mation (including details of support organizations) may help patients to prepare for this difficult period of time and offer longer-term support (see

Chapter 6 for a consideration of the advantages and disadvantages of support organizations). Specialist outpatient services such as those provided by Outlook (below) can be especially useful.

*Health psychologists and multidisciplinary teams*

Increasingly, multidisciplinary teams (MDT) are being seen as the 'gold standard' form of service provision and the one with the most potential to provide a consistent and comprehensive package of care. While some of the support and interventions outlined above could be implemented by any member of an MDT, others (one-to-one interventions) should be offered by specialist psychologists, although currently there are very few health or clinical psychologists offering a designated service for people who have appearance-related concerns. This is despite evidence that adjustment to life changes following health problems, including altered body image, has been identified as being the highest unmet psychological need in a large teaching hospital (Hutton and Williams 2001).

The benefits of having a chartered health psychologist working as part of an MDT and routinely seeing all patients are enormous and have been demonstrated by the success of pain management MDTs where psychologists work alongside medical, nursing and physiotherapy staff to provide an integrated programme of care for patients who share the same symptoms rather than the same aetiology of disease. The model places a firm emphasis on the management of symptoms where their removal is not possible. In essence, how to manage life with an appearance that is different to the norm as opposed to putting life on hold until appearance has been 'corrected'. Perhaps the major advantage of an inclusive approach is the lessening of stigma and uncertainty surrounding referral for psychosocial support. Clarke suggests that many patients refuse referral because they do not understand exactly what is being offered and this is often poorly explained.

A second benefit of having a psychologist within the MDT is their ability to educate and train other members of the team about psychosocial aspects of appearance. Clarke and Cooper (2001) found that specialist nurses working in burn care and head and neck cancer felt they were in a good position to provide support but felt ill equipped and lacked the training to do so (see Chapter 6). This was further supported by Rumsey et al.'s (2004) audit of service provision in clinics in London and Bristol. However, Clarke (2001) demonstrated that head and neck nurse specialists were able to provide appropriate input for patients if adequately resourced and trained. Furthermore, patients reported significant benefits. These findings have encouraged the development of psychosocial training for nurses currently working in relevant areas. A relatively simple one-day training course and supporting resource pack has been found to significantly improve specialist nurses' perceived ability to meet the specific needs of head and neck cancer patients, in particular through the promotion of coping strategies to be used in social situations (Clarke and Cooper 2001). Such training, which can be developed and delivered by health psychologists, represents an efficient means of passing information on to other health care professionals since staff who are trained and experienced in caring for patients with an altered appearance can then play a role in educating other members of the team.

Joint discussions within an MDT also offers the benefit to health care professionals of raising their awareness of the perspectives of other disciplines such as speech and language therapists, physiotherapists, dieticians, dentists and social workers. However, the way in which the multidisciplinary team operates has the potential for problems as well as benefits. For example, a joint consultation in which the patient meets with a large range of health care professionals has been compared to a 'goldfish bowl' and can be a daunting and intimidating experience for the patient (Hearst and Middleton 1997), especially so if that individual finds social and group situations stressful. The anxieties associated with this set-up could be alleviated through the introduction of a patient advocacy model, whereby the patient and family are first seen by a senior member of the team who then acts as an advocate in the team consultation, supporting the patient's efforts to express their problems and seek clarification more easily. The advocate can also check the patient's understanding of the conclusions of the consultation after the event. Alternatively, patients can have individual sessions with team members followed by the MDT meeting for a group discussion afterwards.

Within any multidisciplinary team, health care professionals' own attitudes and beliefs about appearance and disfigurement issues may impact upon their interaction with patients through a variety of ways. For example, they may make assumptions about individuals' reactions to changes in their appearance or their preferences for treatment (Lockhart 1999). Attitudes may also be expressed through the language used in encounters with patients. People with psoriasis have reported being told by their doctors that they should 'just get used' to the disease (Rapp et al. 1997). This was perceived as reflecting the professionals' lack of control over the disease (there remains no cure for psoriasis) but also served to reduce the patients' own sense of control. In contrast, it has been suggested (Tanner et al. 1998) that even when health care staff are unsure as to how a condition will develop and the effect it may have on a patient's appearance (for example in the case of haemangioma) it is still beneficial to provide emotional support and reassurance that they have up-to-date expertise and knowledge about the condition. Health psychologists are well placed to provide support and communication skills training to staff to enable them to deal more effectively with such uncertainties.

*Specialist nursing staff*

Increasingly, specialist nursing staff with advanced training in psychosocial care and counselling skills are being recognized as key members of multi-disciplinary teams, for example within cancers (notably breast cancer, head and neck cancer). A recent development has been the provision of a small number of specialist breast reconstruction nurses who offer a very useful link between consultant plastic surgeons and women contemplating reconstructive surgery. However, this is a very limited service and relatively few women will have access to such specialist support and the continued funding of such posts is rarely guaranteed. The possibilities for the expansion of specialist nursing roles into other appearance-related conditions such as burns and clefts are immense and would be a very welcome addition to the current provision of care.

*Problem-focused psychological support*

Some patients may need support with particular problems at any stage in their treatment. For example, if expectations of outcome are particularly unrealistic, if they appear to be excessively anxious or unclear about treatment options and outcomes. Flashbacks of trauma may be a recurring feature, sometimes as part of post-traumatic stress disorder (PTSD). Long-term follow-up may uncover a failure to re-engage in day-to-day activities, social avoidance and isolation, poor compliance with treatment (for example use of pressure garments), or for children, school refusal or failure. Traditionally, mental health professionals (for example clinical psychologists) have provided the provision of problem-focused psychological support warranted in such situations and the need for this specialist intervention will continue.

Integrating routine and problem-focused support is important in creating a system of comprehensive care. However, a problem-focused approach is only as good as the screening process that identifies problems in the first place. Too often, teams that lack an awareness of psychosocial issues will wait until problems have become 'full blown' – being reactive rather than proactive. While problem-focused support provided by trained psychologists is invaluable, ideally it should be provided by professionals with particular expertise in appearance concerns.

**Specialist services**

Currently, only a small minority of patients identified as needing additional psychosocial support are referred to specialist services offering expert help for individuals with appearance concerns. Most specialist interventions tackle the key difficulties with social encounters through social interaction skills training (SIST) and/or cognitive behavioural therapy (CBT). These have been found to be effective in developing a repertoire of positive coping strategies for managing social situations and the cognitive re-evaluation of appearance as a general commodity rather than as an individual attribute. For example Kleve et al. (2002) stress the benefits of encouraging people with appearance concerns to place less importance on their looks as a component of self-worth and to develop a broader perspective of the self. This fits with the model of adjustment offered in Chapter 2, further suggesting that such a framework could be a workable and useful tool for health care professionals.

Ultimately, services aim to equip individuals with a toolbox of coping strategies to enable them to deal more effectively with the challenges they face. However, despite evidence supporting the use of SIST and CBT, it is important to remember that these approaches will not suit everyone and the possibility of alternative interventions such as person-centred counselling should be considered.

We now consider social interaction skills training (SIST) and cognitive behavioural therapy (CBT) interventions in turn.

*Social interaction skills training*

Social interaction skills training (SIST) involves facilitating an individual's confidence and proficiency around meeting, forming and continuing relationships with other people and has proven effective among a range of patient populations including adolescents affected by a cleft (Kapp-Simon 1995) or burns (Blakeney et al. 1990). Robinson et al. (1996) reported that SIST led to a reduction in social anxiety and avoidance and significant clinical change in 64 clients with a variety of disfigurements. Interventions included role playing, modelling, instruction, feedback and discussions in groups of six to ten individuals on two separate days in order to give participants a chance to practise the skills they had learned between sessions. Reported satisfaction was high, with 73 per cent stating that they would attend future workshops. However, this desire for further input could also indicate that they had not achieved all they had hoped for within the time available. Furthermore, while this combined package was very useful it is still unclear precisely which aspects of such complex interventions are effective. This will take time but should be a focus of future research. One problem is that existing SIST seems to have focused on adults and there is very little research evidence of evaluation of SIST for children and adolescents (Kish and Lansdown 2000).

*Cognitive behavioural therapy*

The principles of CBT have been the mainstay of many interventions for those individuals troubled by their appearance. The available evidence supports the delivery of brief problem-focused CBT interventions rather than longer, costly forms of therapy. For example, Papadopoulos et al.

(1999a) evaluated a CBT programme for vitiligo patients compared with a waiting list control group. The intervention consisted of eight one-hour sessions involving CBT plus teaching of practical skills to help counter negative social attention (staring, coping with comments). The programme led to significant improvements in body image, self-esteem and quality of life that were maintained at follow-up five months later. Papadopoulos and colleagues concluded that this was an especially good intervention since it took place over the summer when the possibilities for effective camouflage are reduced and vitiligo can be particularly stressful. The intervention was also found to have a positive effect on the progression of the disease as evidenced by a reported improvement in pre- and post-intervention photographs of the 12 participants who were not on medication during the intervention. However, this was a small-scale study with only 16 participants in total (eight control, eight intervention) and further evaluations are therefore needed.

*'Outlook' – specialist disfigurement support unit*

Both SIST and CBT have been used within the specialist interventions provided by Outlook, the first designated disfigurement support unit within the NHS which was set up in 1997, at Frenchay Hospital in Bristol. Kleve et al. (2002) discussed the impact of this service in managing appearance-related issues for individuals from a representative hospital population as opposed to just through a support organization focusing specifically on disfigurement. The outcomes of their evaluation are very interesting. Of particular note is the mean number of treatment sessions (n = 3) in delivering a measurable change. Furthermore, many individuals only needed one consultation with a specialist psychologist. Kleve et al.'s evaluation found that the interventions offered by Outlook were helpful in reducing general and social anxiety, appearance-related distress and depressive symptoms, use of camouflage and avoidance as coping strategies. Participants also reported improvements in positive wellbeing, satisfaction with life, social confidence and perceptions of social support, and self-perceptions and perceptions of the noticeability of their disfigurement to other people.

This is an important and cost-effective service. Although the level of intervention reported by Kleve et al. (2002) seems remarkably low, it is supported by evidence from Robinson et al.'s (1996) evaluation of a relatively brief, social interaction skills workshops for people with a facial disfigurement.

A specialist outpatient service such as Outlook is particularly appropriate since many of the problems experienced by individuals will only be encountered once they have left the relative security of a hospital environment (Kleve and Robinson 1999). Outlook offers interventions on individual, one-to-one and group bases. While group interventions offer a more economic means of delivering interventions, it has been suggested that patients prefer individual to group therapy (Fortune 1998; Kleve and Robinson 1999) possibly because their anxieties surrounding social encounters render the concept of group meetings additionally challenging. A combined, flexible approach offering individual therapy in the first instance in order to increase social confidence and reduce social anxiety might then enable an individual to benefit from a group intervention (see Chapter 6).

The work conducted by Outlook has demonstrated that the conceptual framework of 'disfigurement' *per se* (see Chapter 2) is useful in a specialized, clinical context. Yet it is important to remember that a highly specialist service will not be able to address all of an individual's problems. Kleve et al. (2002) found that the appearance–specific intervention offered by Outlook was most beneficial to a sub-set of clients whose distress was specifically related to appearance as opposed to a range of other additional difficulties.

Outlook's work includes supporting children through the transition from primary to secondary school since this can be an anxiety-provoking time. A summer programme for children and adults normalizes the experience of school transition, recognizing that all children have concerns about making new friends, leaving the familiarity of one school for the uncertainty of another (which is often much larger) and also from being one of the senior members of a school to being one of the youngest. Again, the non–condition specific programme involves CBT and focuses on problem-solving activities to tackle teasing during a half-day intervention and follow-up after the transition to the new school has taken place. A low–scale evaluation of this brief intervention to date has reported it as being cheap and effective (Maddern and Owen 2004). Further evaluation of the unit's intervention with children (50 per cent of whom had a craniofacial condition such as a cleft) has demonstrated a reduction in the frequency of teasing and the degree of distress caused by their appearance in school or in the playground (Maddern and Emerson 2002). They also reported statistically significant reductions in parental reports of their children's problems, particularly somatizing behaviour, withdrawal and anxiety.

The problem with the current provision of specialist services is that they are not available to all and are likely only to be taken up by those with the ability and time to travel. Services need to be practically and logistically available. Maddern and Owen (2004) report how the Outlook summer school transfer programme is run on a single day to make it more accessible for families who would be unable to travel considerable distances for a series of hour–long sessions. Similarly, Hughes (1998) suggests that guidance offered by the Disfigurement Guidance Centre in Fife, Scotland will only be accessed by particularly motivated individuals who are prepared and able to travel. This also means that research conducted in scarce specialist centres is potentially biased, since only those who are sufficiently able or committed to travelling for the intervention will be included. It was hoped that Robinson et al.'s and Kleve et al.'s positive evaluations would result in Outlook being spread across the UK. However, limited financial resources being directed towards specialist services such as this or within the field of disfigurement more generally have prevented this from occurring, with the resulting reliance upon the voluntary sector.

### New possibilities

One of the many interesting challenges for psychologists working in this field is the development of new effective methods of providing psychosocial support and interventions for the large numbers of people with appearance-related concerns, with or without a visible difference. A consideration of interventions currently available among other populations is an obvious starting point in the search for ideas. For example, one of the perceived drawbacks of traditional CBT has been the cost of psychological input. However, self-directed CBT (for example Cash's *Body Image Workbook* – see Chapter 6) has been effective among people with body dissatisfaction, and evaluations of web-based interventions (Beat the Blues, a programme for people suffering from depression) suggest that the Internet has great potential for cost-effective and accessible delivery of CBT-based interventions.

Another interesting possibility is the use of written emotional expression. Spending a designated period of time writing about a particularly stressful event has proven beneficial in terms of improved psychological wellbeing (see Bennett (2004) for a brief overview). Hamilton-West and Bridle (2004) found that written emotional disclosure following a fire in a student hall of residence significantly increased health status as assessed by the GHQ, possibly because the intervention had overridden spontaneous, ineffective coping efforts. In this instance, none of the participants had suffered burn injuries and this type of intervention has yet to be tested in a clinical population with appearance issues. While this would be an interesting avenue to pursue, caution is warranted since participants could be at risk of PTSD and such interventions might encourage some individuals to ruminate on their difficulties and encourage maladaptive coping strategies rather than benefit from disclosing their concerns. Cameron and Nicholls (1998) suggest that written emotional disclosure interventions structured around self-regulation theory, and including the writing of a coping plan which is subsequently appraised and revised, may be more useful for those with optimistic tendencies. Furthermore, the impact of writing about positive aspects and thoughts about one's appearance and focusing on what has helped an individual might be beneficial, as opposed to an exclusive focus on the difficulties and stresses encountered.

## School-based interventions for those with a visible difference

Much of the specialist support for adults and children with a visible difference is provided by the voluntary sector. Most referrals (30.9 per cent) to the charity Changing Faces are triggered by a pupil with a visible difference attending a new school (Frances 2000). The Changing Faces schools service offers expert advice and specially developed services for teachers, early-years workers and educational professionals supporting children and teenagers with disfigurements. This is necessary because it is difficult for teachers and educational professionals to gain experience and expertise since, despite the widespread nature of appearance-related concerns, most schools will only occasionally have a pupil with a visible difference. An educational package including materials designed by Changing Faces has been shown to raise primary school children's awareness of their attitudes and behaviours towards facial appearance and improve the reception they give to people with a visible disfigurement (Cline et al. 1998).

However, given the incidence of appearance concerns in the general adolescent population (see Chapter 3) it seems likely that all school staff are in contact with students with appearance concerns and therefore warrant training and support. (See the research by Lovegrove and Rumsey (2005) outlined earlier.) It could also be argued that a similar situation exists in other professions and working environments. Indeed, Changing Faces have developed educative approaches and materials for employers and produced condition-specific information packs and training courses for health care professionals working with those who are visibly different.

Regarding school-based support for children with a visible difference, Frances (2000) stresses the need for all those concerned (for example child, family, key staff) to reach agreement over what is considered important for others to know and who should be told (teaching staff only, all pupils and so on). Depending on the age of the child, he or she should also be involved in these decisions.

One challenge facing any specialist intervention, be it school based or otherwise, is how to avoid unwittingly overemphasizing one person's difference and by default exaggerating everyone else's homogeneity. Rather the aim should be to encourage acceptance and diversity. For example, the Outlook summer camp (Maddern and Owen 2004) acknowledges that all children have concerns about starting at a new school, yet clearly the challenges facing a child with a visible difference will, in some respects, differ from those facing other children.

## Towards a comprehensive system of care

A comprehensive system of care requires support being made available across the lifespan and, where appropriate, at all stages of treatment. Failure to do so could be seen as encouraging the belief, highlighted in Chapter 2, that appearance is always a concern for adolescents and not for older people. Currently, the limited research among cleft palate patients for example has focused on children and adolescents, with a dearth of studies and interventions focusing on adults, yet the psychosocial challenges may persist throughout adulthood (Elmendorf et al. 1993; Robinson 1997; see also Chapter 4). Comprehensive psychosocial support may also benefit physical aspects of some conditions. For example, stress management interventions may be helpful for individuals with conditions such as psoriasis which are believed to be exacerbated by stress (Fortune et al. 2005; Rapp et al. 1997).

Interventions should not only focus on the individual who has concerns about their appearance. Rather, they should be available to family members and to the wider community through sociocultural and media interventions. In Chapter 4 we discussed issues relating to the provision of care for parents when a child is prenatally diagnosed or born with a visible difference. The Outlook Disfigurement Support Unit offers support for parents alongside that provided for children (Maddern and Owen 2004). Running the group alongside the children's sessions has encouraged the development of a positive group for parents, yet the unit suggests that fathers are under-represented. This may be due to practical and logistical reasons or it may indicate that they find it harder than mothers to accept such support. In response to these concerns, a group specifically for fathers is being established in the hope that this will appeal to them more.

One of the major benefits of clinical services organized in voluntary settings is the opportunity for the client to remain in control. Organizations such as Changing Faces accept referrals directly without the need to consult a GP. Referrals to health care services involve waiting times and screening processes, and the problem often becomes medically framed at the outset: psychosocial intervention is offered less as a valid alternative and more as a second best if medical intervention is ineffective. In an ideal world both voluntary and health care sectors will benefit from close collaboration and the development of new and innovative ways of providing psychosocial care.

One final area for consideration is the topic of lay-led self-management, recently promoted in the UK as part of the 'Expert Patient Programme'. This radical new idea, pioneered by Lorig et al. (1999) trains service users to deliver a structured course for people living with a chronic illness. Characterized by information giving and the development of personal action planning, these courses are run by non-health professionals and can be effective in promoting self-efficacy, a sense of control and providing the skills needed to manage their condition to complement existing health care provision (see Cooper and Clarke (2001) for the Long-Term Medical Condition Alliance (LMCA)). Changing Faces was one of the first examples of an effective lay-led self-management programme in the UK. While the need for lay-led self-management programmes to be supported by credible, evidence-based evaluation has been stated (Clarke and Cooper 2001), its full potential is yet to be investigated.

## Conclusion

There is increasing interest in the provision of psychosocial care not only as an adjunct to biomedical interventions, but increasingly as an alternative. Biomedical interventions are increasingly recognized by those delivering them as only a partial answer to complex problems. However, it is important to remember that not everyone will want support to cope with appearance-related issues. Kent and Keohane (2001) conclude that the demand for assistance might come from those whose condition is visible and whose fear of negative evaluation is high. A combination of social skills training and cognitive behavioural therapy appears to be an effective package but confidence in the potential for more effective support and intervention is directly related to the quality of the available evidence base. This is an important focus for the next generation of research studies.

Ideally in years to come, appearance will be a recognized and legitimate issue within many systems of care. The bulk of these concerns could be addressed through routine care provided by health care professionals, while those individuals requiring more detailed support should be able to access appropriate services easily through the health care or voluntary sector. Health psychologists have a key role to play in this respect, from training and supporting health care staff to providing specialist support and evaluating the effectiveness of care provision at all levels.

Increased funding is needed both for research and for psychosocial care and support in order that it can be readily available and provided proactively rather than merely as a reaction. Furthermore, a more positive approach towards appearance requires a change in attitudes. To this end, the media and school-based interventions have a significant contribution to make.

## Chapter summary

♦ The potential for improving the provision of support and interventions for people with appearance-related concerns is considerable. Health psychologists have a valuable role to play in this process;
♦ The power of the media through the advertising industry and television could be used to promote acceptance of diversity of appearance;
♦ Many people engage in health behaviours because of the impact they have on appearance rather than their anticipated health benefits. Health promotion campaigns could make greater use of this concern with appearance, but must be wary not to reinforce beauty myths and stereotypes;

♦ While very few interventions aim at tackling appearance-related concerns among people without a visible difference, school-based interventions for young people and appearance dissatisfaction treatment programmes have a great deal of potential;

♦ Appearance should be recognized as a legitimate concern within any health care situation, not only those catering specifically for people with a visible difference;

♦ Ideally, psychosocial support for people with visible differences is provided through a combination of general support as part of routine care and specific interventions to help those identified as having particular concerns;

♦ All health care staff have a role to play to providing comprehensive care for people with a visible difference and those around them. This may require appropriate staff training and support;

♦ Specialist interventions have tended to focus on social interactions skills training and cognitive behavioural therapy and have been found beneficial;

♦ Ideally, specialist disfigurement support centres would be more widely available than is currently the case;

♦ There is much potential for the development of new and innovative psychosocial interventions in this area.

## Discussion points

♦ How might you go about trying to influence societal attitudes towards disfigurement?

♦ How could health psychologists influence the provision of care for people with appearance-related concerns?

♦ To what extent do you agree with the suggestion that people should be persuaded to pay less attention to their image and more to their health?

## Further reading

Clarke, A. (1999) Psychosocial aspects of facial disfigurement: problems, management and the role of a lay-led organization. *Psychology, Health and Medicine*, 4: 128–41.

Newell, R. (2000) *Body Image and Disfigurement Care*. London: Routledge.

# Conclusions, dilemmas and the challenges still ahead

In this book we have offered a synthesis and critical review of research and an overview of care provision relating to the psychological aspects of appearance. The fascination humans have with appearance is nothing new. People have been interested and investing in their appearance for centuries. However, what is new is the acknowledgement of the ramifications of appearance concerns for those affected, a growing appreciation of the complexity of the factors involved in adjustment and a progression away from the previously exclusive focus on issues of weight and body image.

As researchers who originally concentrated their attention on the negative experiences of people with visible differences, we now appreciate that appearance is also a source of concern and distress for a sizeable proportion of the population whose appearance to others is ostensibly 'normal'. Issues such as social anxiety and self-consciousness are commonly reported by many individuals regardless of whether or not they have an unusual appearance. It is likely that these people would also benefit from appropriate psychosocial support but unfortunately health care provision to meet the needs of those affected typically falls short of the ideal. A proportion of people with or without a visible difference demonstrate positive adjustment to appearance issues, and researchers and clinicians have much still to learn from these individuals.

## Challenges ahead

There are several challenges ahead for appearance researchers, including raising awareness of the importance of studying the psychology of appearance; promoting a positive agenda for appearance research and care provision; improving health care services; developing theory and research; changing attitudes towards appearance and informing and contributing to the debates around current dilemmas including the impact of new computer technologies on norms of physical attractiveness and the challenges posed by advances in screening, genetic and transplantation technologies.

### Raising awareness of the importance of understanding and studying appearance

We hope that, by now, readers are convinced that appearance is both a legitimate and important concern for health psychologists and others concerned with optimizing health and wellbeing. Concerns about appearance can influence a wide range of health behaviours, including for example diet and exercise. Given that these are currently central to UK Government health policy, it would be shortsighted to ignore the evidence that appearance underpins many aspects of health behaviour change. Appearance issues can also influence health care decision making and adherence to treatment, for example when treatment or its side effects have an actual or perceived impact on the way we look.

Given the pervasive nature of appearance concerns and the far-reaching ramifications of these issues, we hope to see appearance included in academic and practitioner training programmes. The opportunities that involvement in appearance-related research and interventions offers health psychologists in both clinical and research settings are many, varied, challenging and rewarding.

### Promoting a positive agenda towards appearance

Having focused in the past on pathology and negative experiences of appearance (for example psychological distress and body dissatisfaction) the time has now come to foster a broader approach. In recent years, repeated calls have been made for a more positive agenda for people living with an unusual appearance since systems of health care provision based only on problems and difficulties do little to promote positive adjustment to visible difference (see Chapter 6). Researchers and clinicians have much to contribute to the recent calls for society to celebrate diversity in appearance, rather than pander slavishly to the ever more exacting 'ideals' handed out through the media. However, we are also aware that we need to guard against overzealousness in our enthusiasm for the agenda of positive adjustment, as overemphasizing the virtues of resilience to appearance concerns could result in those affected feeling a burden to cope positively, and make them less able to voice concerns about their difficulties.

### Improving the provision of care

It seems inevitable that increasing numbers of people will seek some kind of support or intervention in relation to dissatisfaction and concerns relating to their appearance. This is likely to include a continued rise in the number of people seeking cosmetic surgical and non-surgical procedures. Harris and Carr (2001) articulated the need for well-regulated surgical and psychological services for people with problems of appearance in both the NHS and independent sectors. It is clear that health psychologists have the skills and knowledge needed to influence the provision of such care in a variety of ways.

While surgeons continue to develop new technologies with the potential to improve quality of life for many people with appearance concerns, it is vital that the psychosocial implications of these developments are carefully examined. The potential role for health psychologists in the introduction of these supposed advances is considerable, for example in the provision of appropriate, accurate information about the risks and benefits of procedures, in supporting decision making, and in researching outcomes.

Another important role for health and clinical psychologists is to train and support health care professionals to recognize the pervasiveness and impact of appearance concerns. Working at grassroots level, to demonstrate and persuade health care professionals of the ramifications of these issues is arguably the most effective way of improving care for those affected. In reality, the extent to which journal publications influence care provision is dubious. Raising awareness of these issues in conditions that have previously been considered only in terms of function such as eye problems (Clarke et al. 2003) should be a priority and would facilitate an ethos of care in which appearance is recognized as an important issue within any health care situation. To this end we support Pruzinsky's (2004) call for body image/ appearance assessment to become part of routine care (see Chapter 6). The recent requirement for all cleft care teams in the UK to include an appropriately trained psychologist has been an exciting development. Having set a precedent, this is a standard of care that would ideally be extended to other specialities and conditions.

Clear referral routes are needed for those individuals identified as warranting additional psychosocial support and specialist interventions. Ideally, these would be provided by specialist staff through a national network of specialist centres. However, given the lack of dedicated resources, there is a need to investigate alternative options including new interventions and technology. The Internet offers the potential for new methods of easily accessible information and intervention that have yet to be explored fully in this context (see Chapter 7).

As well as working directly with health care professionals delivering care, one of the most effective ways in which psychologists can exert an influence is by engaging with policy makers who effectively shape systems of care. Two ways of doing this are first, to ensure that research findings are clearly disseminated to audiences of policy makers and second, to engage with relevant forums in which aspects of care provision, including appearance issues are discussed. UK regulation of the cosmetic surgery industry formed part of the 5th Report of the House of Commons Select Committee on Health. This report criticized the pressures put on consumers by commercially operated clinics in the private sector who at that time were not governed by strict controls. Under UK guidelines proposed in January 2005, the cosmetic surgery industry (including the administration of botox injections, implants and chemical skin peels) will be subject to a number of regulations aiming to raise standards and protect prospective patients from unqualified, unregistered practitioners, misleading advertisements and inadequate information about possible side effects and complications. The success and impact of these regulations on the experiences and wellbeing of people seeking private cosmetic surgery remains to be seen.

### Changing attitudes towards appearance

Our expectations of attractiveness are, thanks to the media and the increasing availability of appearance-altering treatments, constantly escalating. Yet we seem to be living through an epidemic of body dissatisfaction and discontent with our appearance (see Chapters 3 and 4). Sadly, many of the dissatisfied people use their appearance as a hook on which to hang their problems, and come to believe their lives would be much better if only they looked differently. The continual growth of the fashion, cosmetics and private surgery industries reflects the lengths to which some people will go in order to try to attain an ideal, yet probably unachievable, appearance. Others are far less susceptible to the messages portrayed by these industries and through the media, and while research is starting to explore these individual differences this is an area with much potential for future research. Changing attitudes towards appearance is a difficult yet necessary task if the trend towards dissatisfaction is to be reversed and society is to become more accepting of a diversity of appearances. Efforts at changing societal attitudes could do much to improve the quality of life of people whose appearance concerns and perceived inability to meet society's exacting standards are a source of distress and unhappiness but will need to involve individuals, health care professionals, policy makers, voluntary organizations, industry, media, researchers and schools.

### Developing theory and research

Existing theories aiming to explain and understand individuals' experiences of their appearance have been of limited use due to their tendency to focus on a pathological approach and because of the myriad of complex factors likely to play a role in determining adjustment to appearance (see Chapter 2). These include cognitive and emotional responses, family environment, peer values, the responses of others, the sociocultural context, actual physical appearance and developmental stage. An integrative, predictive and testable framework that relates to people with or without a visible difference and allows for a focus on positive experiences as well as problems and difficulties would provide a more cohesive conceptual basis than has previously been the case and would offer clear guidance for clinical application and the provision of evidence-based care. Such research evidence is likely to be pieced together from a variety of sources with researchers needing to employ a range of methods and methodologies.

Appearance will continue to be a challenging and engaging area for health psychology researchers (see Chapter 2). In summary, there is a need for research that is longitudinal, includes both positive and negative aspects of appearance and takes full advantage of the wide range of methods that are at our disposal. There is a pressing need for research to include a broader range of population groups, specifically those from a wider range of ethnic and cultural groups and drawn from across the lifespan. Research is also needed to influence thinking about initiatives relating to the provision of care, for example the development of new disciplines such as oncoplastics (combining cancer and plastic surgery) and psychodermatology and in relation to the introduction of new technologies and procedures.

Rather than ending this book in the time-honoured way with our conclusions, we have chosen to offer readers a selection of dilemmas that are currently taxing us and that offer a wealth of opportunities for input of health psychologists and other appearance researchers in the future.

## Current dilemmas

For those who enjoy grappling with ethical and moral dilemmas, the domain of appearance research contains some interesting challenges. We live in an age where there are decreasing levels of tolerance of the physical manifestations of nature and our genetic inheritance. Adults and even children now use cosmetic surgery, orthodontics, exercise, diet and lifestyle drugs in attempts to match up to the perfect physiques and allegedly happy lives depicted in the media, eagerly embracing new appearance-enhancing techniques as they come on stream.

Rapidly developing new technologies present some particularly interesting challenges and dilemmas including those which at face value may seem exciting, and which may offer considerable potential benefits. As is the case with other recent developments in health care, the psychological benefits of new technologies have been assumed although the actual impact is much less certain and is likely to be much more complex than policy makers and providers of health care assume.

The following developments will be considered as exemplars. First, the impact of recent technologies on norms of physical appearance and attractiveness, and second, three examples specifically relevant to health care provision: prenatal screening and the diagnosis of clefts; genetic engineering and the concept of 'designer babies'; and lastly, the imminent possibility of whole face transplantation.

## The impact of technology on norms of physical attractiveness

Advances in computer technology have made it possible in recent years to produce 'virtual' faces, which may be composites of the 'best' features of more than one face, or generated entirely by computer. This technology has been greeted with considerable enthusiasm and clearly has some worthwhile applications, including enhanced techniques to facilitate eye witness testimony and identification together with other forensic techniques such as the more accurate modelling of facial appearance from skeletal structures. In addition, plastic surgeons are excited by the possibility of adapting digital technology and software developed by the film industry (which permit the substitution of computer-generated images as stunt doubles in films and to enhance or replace aspects of an actor's appearance through digital imagery) to demonstrate the likely post-operative outcome following an aesthetic or reconstructive surgical procedure.

3D computer animations are now being widely used in games and animation cartoons. Avatars (computerized figures or images used to represent real people), most famously Lara Croft from the game *Tomb Raider*, are created and regularly enhanced to incorporate an ever-wider range of behavioural and emotional expressions, and are used to role play and interact on line. Applications of these technologies in other media are also becoming more pervasive. Digital models have begun to appear on TV adverts, in films and on mobile phones. Britain's first virtual newscaster was launched on the Internet in 2000: 'Ananova has been programmed to deliver the news in a "pleasant, quietly intelligent manner" and is designed to portray the characteristics of a single 28-year-old, attractive "girl about town" who loves Oasis, the Simpsons and is 5'8" tall' (Kemp et al. 2004: 135). In Japan, digital models have been used to sell a range of products, from computers to cosmetics to cash loans. Japan's first virtual pop star hit the charts in Tokyo as long ago as 1996.

Kemp and colleagues (2004) report that in 2003, digital artists from around the world were invited to send a computer design of their 'perfect' woman, complete with measurements for the Internet beauty content 'Digital Miss World'. They also reported a study in which researchers offered a selection of real and composite faces to a model agency. Fourteen out of the 16 chosen as most likely to succeed were unreal composites. Are the model faces and bodies of the future going to follow the trend set by Barbie (see Chapter 3) and become still less attainable? The answer would seem to be 'yes', but there is a twist! Beauty has long been thought to be underpinned by symmetry. Computer technology now allows us to measure this and to find the most symmetrical faces (or make composite faces). However, as Kemp and colleagues (2004) point out in relation to these composites 'there is something almost sinister about the uniformity of a very symmetrical face – those with less symmetry appear more full of life'. They note that interestingly, some have begun to model in 'imperfections', such as freckles, bushy eyebrows, chipped or uneven teeth. Others are going for perfection – though some judge the more perfect as lifelessness (Kemp et al. 2004), especially with regard to the eyes and plasticity of the face. As Kemp and colleagues say: 'how ironic it would be if the siren call to perfection were to flatten the very diversity we need to be human'.

Somewhat comfortingly, although digital artists are succeeding in producing ever-more beautiful 'still' faces, animators are experiencing considerable difficulties in producing realistic moving faces through computer animation. The naturalness of the face depends on intricate movements and also complex timing. A smile can be natural only if spontaneity is maintained and the animation of all parts of the face is perfectly synchronized. This is particularly apparent in the eyes, and in a lack of plasticity in the face.

We wait to see what the psychological impact of images of faces and bodies no longer shaped by biology alone, but progressively engineered through new technologies will be. Will the distress and dissatisfaction of those who are unhappy with the way they look now be increased by ever-more unattainable images, or might these images become sufficiently removed from reality to cease to offer a credible standard of comparison?

### New technologies in the context of health care

#### Advances in antenatal screening

Recent advances in antenatal screening technologies mean that increasing numbers of congenital impairments affecting appearance are identified before birth. The most common of these is a cleft of the lip (see Chapter 4). Although legal terminations after 24 weeks gestation can only be carried out in the case of 'severe foetal abnormality', the interpretation of 'severe' is left to physicians and parents. A recent legal challenge in the UK was brought by Jepson, an Anglican curate, who argued against the termination of the pregnancy of a foetus with a cleft lip on the grounds that this should not be classed as a 'severe abnormality'. Clefts are not life threatening. In westernized countries, they are surgically corrected within the first six months of life, although treatment (including speech therapy, treatment for hearing deficits, orthodontic treatment and surgery to the lip, nose and upper jaw) can be required throughout childhood and adolescence. Approximately 20–35 per cent of those born with a cleft are thought to experience psychological difficulties at some point in their development, but the majority do well (see Chapter 4). As Strauss (2001) pointed out, clefts can be treated, and are certainly not a barrier to a rich and fulfilling life. However, Jepson's case brought into sharp relief the importance attached to physical appearance and the lengths prospective parents are prepared to go to achieve a 'perfect' baby. In addition, the financial burden of initial and ongoing treatment in countries with state-funded health care such as the USA, can be considerable, and levels of insurance and income can be an additional factor affecting the decision parents make about whether or not to continue with a pregnancy.

The expertise of health psychologists could usefully be applied in this domain of antenatal screening. Although for some a routine scan provides reassuring information, for others, especially those for whom the outcome is not all good news, this type of screening can be a burden. It may certainly become increasingly difficult for women who prefer not to have this information prior to the birth to feel they can step off the screening conveyor belt and decline to have the tests, as screening can enhance the chances of a successful outcome to the pregnancy. If an impairment is identified, the need to take the decision of whether to end or continue with a wanted pregnancy is likely to be associated with major guilt and distress (see Chapter 4), especially if the condition is not life threatening.

The high termination rates reported in the USA have led health care professionals and psychologists in the UK to consider who is the most appropriate person to provide information to parents following the positive identification of a cleft, and also, what information should be offered. Good practice guidelines in the UK now recommend that a cleft team member (often the surgeon) contacts the parents within 24 hours of the diagnosis, and that care is taken to offer the parents clear and balanced information about the treatment options. As psychologists are currently being appointed as core cleft team members in the UK (see Chapter 6), it is likely that they will play an increasingly key role in the provision of information and ongoing support.

In addition, the impact of increasing numbers of terminations on the many people already living with a treated cleft must be considered. The debate about whether or not such an infant is viewed as 'flawed', or with a 'serious abnormality' will impact on them too. They may feel that their own life has been devalued and may need support.

*Advances in genetic engineering ('designer babies')*

In recent years, excitement about the mapping of the human genome has led to speculation about the potential applications of gene therapy. Those in favour of genetic engineering focus on the potential of these technologies to rule out pre-existing impairments, or to counter the disposition to develop serious diseases in later life. However, for the sceptics there is a very thin line between removing impairments and creating designer babies.

In appearance terms, commentators have begun to speculate on the consequences of 'designing' babies to be more beautiful. Some argue that this would be an appropriate use of genetic engineering, but what might the psychological consequences of creating these 'designer babies' be for the babies themselves, their families and society at large? However, as Pickering (1991) so aptly warned in the context of gene therapy, there is at least a need 'to sound a note of warning of fog further down the line'. Immediate questions come to mind. For example, who should decide what kinds of appearance-related genetic alterations are acceptable? What standards or norms will be used? Will it be permissible for humans to be engineered according to current societal values (Agar 1998)? Is taller better than shorter? Is black hair preferable to blonde? Are blue eyes better than brown? Will there be new classes of inferiority? What becomes the norm – the Barbie Doll, an avatar or Digital Miss World? Through being able to choose to alter appearance in this way, will we become more sensitive to difference and increase our prejudice against it? The experience of the impact of previous appearance-enhancing procedures suggests the answer is likely to be 'yes'. In a broader context, Murphy and Lappe (1994) maintained that the moral significance of the genome project lies in its impact on the interpretation of normalcy and difference.

What will be the impact on the child – in particular his or her sense of identity and self-worth? Will those who have had their gene sequence modified feel they have been altered to match up to the expectations of parents that they would otherwise have fallen short of? Will they be beset by the insecurities reported by some people who rely heavily on their beauty (see Chapter 3), and feel that their parents, friends and lovers only want them if they are beautiful? Will they rely too heavily on their appearance to attract others and fail to invest in other relationship skills? What if appearance norms change over the course of a lifetime, or if their appearance preferences differ from those chosen by their parents? Perhaps they will resent the hair and eye colour their parents 'ordered' with the best of intentions.

What of the impact on parents? How will the physical appearance of the child affect their broader expectations? Do they want their offspring to look more beautiful since they believe this is the key to happiness in life? The evidence to support this assumption is lacking (see Chapter 3). Will they expect that a beautiful personality will accompany the looks, and will they be disappointed to discover this is not necessarily the case? Perhaps they will 'order' a beautiful child as a trophy to be displayed to the world? Warnock (1992) and others have warned that the emphasis on the potential of genetic engineering detracts from the considerable influence of the environment on the development and adjustment of children, adolescents and adults. As the geneticist Lander (1992) said: 'spend more time with your kid; that would make more difference [than tinkering with the gene sequence]'.

As with the introduction of other new ways to alter appearance, there will also be consequences for the millions of people living with an appearance which is considered different from the prevailing norm: the numbers of these people will rise as the definition of normal becomes narrower, and for the millions more who are distressed by the way they look. Diversity in appearance is needed in order to avoid marginalizing those who have an unusual appearance. Above all, what are the consequences of buying into ever-more extreme ways of altering the external manifestations of our ancestral and genetic packaging?

Is it too far-fetched to believe that parents really will go for the option of enhancing appearance through genetic engineering once it exists? The eugenic impulse is strong (Davis 1995). Parents want the best for their children, so given the chance, it is certainly possible they will take it. Appleyard (1999) reported that 11 per cent of Americans said they might abort a child who was found to be predisposed to obesity. Initially, this type of genetic intervention is likely to be the preserve of the affluent, but as Appleyard adds, this is the age of consumerism and vanity – if it can be bought, it will be. If it is possible to make an offspring more beautiful, many will go for it, despite the fact that many commentators feel we should fight the tendency to stigmatize anything that can reasonably be regarded as healthy variation.

*Advances in surgical and immunological techniques*

In a blaze of media attention, surgeons in the USA, the UK and France announced in 2003 that they were ready to perform whole face transplantation. This procedure involves cutting and lifting skin and fat, arteries and veins (and potentially nerves and muscles) from a recently deceased donor and attaching it to a recipient, whose previous facial skin and fat has also been removed. Although the transplant teams involved originally envisaged the procedure as an intervention for those who had been severely disfigured as the result of burns, cancer or extensive trauma, the degree to which the media focused on this angle, and the accuracy of the detail of the risks involved was very variable. In the UK, there was a media frenzy to find the likely first recipient. Public understanding of the risks involved appears patchy – with some akin to the film *Face Off* in which one fully functioning face was swapped (without any signs of surgery) for another!

The initial trumpet blowing surrounding the possibility of face transplantation was reminiscent of the words of Ian Kennedy (1988): 'if you can do it you must do it. The moment you find out that you can do a new operation it must be done regardless of the expense and of the danger and regardless of the availability of safer, simpler, effective and more economic options. Then let other people pick up later the intellectual, legal and moral cat's cradle that you may have left in your wake'. Ward (1999) expanded on Kennedy's thoughts about the technological imperative experienced by surgeons in the context of plastic surgery. He coined the term 'high trapeze surgery' to refer to the desire to walk the surgical tightrope in preference to rejecting new and exciting procedures. A desire which Ward believes can cloud an objective assessment of the perceived benefits and risks for the patient and which may result in surgical procedures which constitute uncontrolled experimentation.

Despite the enthusiasm of the teams involved, the announcements of their readiness to proceed received a mixed reception from professionals and commentators in the countries concerned. In the UK, the Royal College of Surgeons convened an expert group to deliberate on whether this procedure was advisable at the present time. This group concluded that the transplant teams should wait until more is known about the risks both of tissue rejection and the psychological impact on the recipient and donor families (Royal College of Surgeons 2003; see also Morris et al. 2004). In March 2004, after more than two years' deliberation, the French National Ethics Consultative Committee (CCNE) said 'No' to whole face transplantation, describing the procedure as too 'experimental', describing it as 'spectacular' but 'pointless and too risky'. However, surgeons and scientists at the University of Kentucky are continuing to seek ethical approval from their institutional review board (university ethics committee) to carry out these procedures.

The potential psychological consequences of face transplantation are considerable. The unique significance of the face makes it difficult to extrapolate with confidence from the limited literature on the psychological effects of other forms of transplantation, and psychologists are in the difficult position of not being able to study at first hand the consequences of face transplantation until after the procedure has been carried out a reasonable number of times. As with many other forms of appearance-enhancing surgery, the assumptions made by the surgical teams reflect the prevailing biomedical model of care (see Chapter 6), and the underlying assumption that life will only get better is if you look better – hence many psychological benefits of a potentially more 'normal' appearance are assumed. Readers will know by now that the picture is likely to be much more complex than this! Adjustment is not well predicted by the severity of a disfigurement (see Chapter 4). Powerful elements of adjustment include levels of self-esteem (and the extent to which this is derived from qualities other than outward appearance), the quality of a person's support network and the effectiveness of his or her social interaction skills (see Chapter 5). Those who are most distressed by their appearance may be most psychologically vulnerable, and least well equipped to deal with the rigours of complex surgery, uncertain outcomes and demanding post-operative regimes (Rumsey 2004). There may be significant consequences for the recipient, the recipient's family, the donor and the donor's family, together with broader societal consequences. A detailed discussion is beyond the scope of this chapter (interested readers are referred to Morris et al. (2004)), however, the transplant literature, and other research relating to the significance of the face suggest the following should be considered.

Researchers have become increasingly aware that other forms of transplantation can give rise to a particular set of stressors, psychosocial challenges and adaptive demands (Ziegelmann et al. 2002). These include fears relating to the viability and possible rejection of the transplanted organ and the aftermath of rejection; the burden of personal responsibility for the success or failure of the graft arising from the need to adhere to an often complex drug regime; the need to alter some behaviour patterns (for example diet to reduce the risk of post-operative diabetes which occurs in 7–12 per cent of transplant patients and guarding against sun exposure to reduce the risk of skin cancer in view of the compromised immune system). Some degree of non-adherence to post-transplant treatment regimes is surprisingly common, with levels of 15–18 per cent reported in previous studies (Dew et al. 2001). Current estimates are that up to 10 per cent of face transplants will be rejected within the first 12 months post-transplant, and between 30 and 50 per cent will be rejected in the first five years following the initial procedure (Concar 2004). The consequences of rejection are severe, as the only possibilities are to regraft the face with skin taken from the recipient's own body, or to perform a further face transplant.

A further set of anxieties relate to the potential side effects of the immunosuppressive medication, which currently would need to be taken in perpetuity to reduce the risk of rejection of the transplant. These include significant increases in the risk of infections and in most types of malignancy, especially where a viral cause is implicated. If a malignancy did develop, the choice would be to halt immunosuppression with the concomitant risk of the loss of the transplant, or to continue to suppress the immune system and increase the risk of the progression of the malignancy.

Recipients, their families and friends will have to assimilate the new appearance into an existing body image and sense of identity. Will family and friends find it more or less difficult than dealing with a damaged version of the original face? The proposed early recipients of face transplants may favour the prospect of a non-disfigured face to their visibly different one. However, the psychological and social effects of 'wearing' a face that previously fronted an entirely different person is unknown. Previous literature about stress associated with disruption to one's facial appearance, and issues about projecting the 'real me' to others (Bradbury 1997) may well remain. Facial expressions are crucial in our encounters with others. Difficulties with communication are likely to play a part in motivating potential recipients to seek a face transplant. However, the extent to which the new face is likely to function fully after the transplant is unknown. Current estimates are that 50 per cent of full function may be achievable, although facial nerves will take some time to grow back, and this may be an optimistic estimate of final levels of facial functioning (Concar 2004). Non-verbal communication is likely to be compromised and the face may have a mask-like quality resulting from lack of movement. There is a possibility of uncontrolled facial spasms and expressions.

As initial indications are that donors will be few and far between, the potential recipient is likely to have to endure a long wait for a suitable donor.

Will life be put on hold in the meantime, and how will potential recipients cope during the wait with the inevitable anxieties about their eventual post-operative appearance (Rumsey 2004)? How close will the match be in relation to gender, age, skin colour and tone? Will recipients wish and/or be permitted any choice in relation to the potential donor face?

Recipients will have to deal with the reactions of friends and family both to an altered appearance and changes in familiar patterns of expression and non-verbal communication. The responses from others to a new face will be different, even if only in subtle ways. Some degree of mismatch between the recipient's pre-operative expectations and the actual reactions of others is likely. It is also likely that intrusive media coverage will surround the first face transplants.

Although there is little research to date relating to the impact of transplant on recipients' families, and donor families, psychosocial support is likely to be both necessary and beneficial. Along with the recipients, their families may find the wait for a donor stressful. Support may also be required with acceptance of the altered post-operative appearance of the family member, with efforts to maximize levels of adherence to post-operative treatment regimes and in relation to early face transplant procedures, the pressures of intensive media coverage. The motivation of donor families to donate a face should be carefully explored. Do they expect their loved one to live on in some way? Will they want to contact the recipient? Even if the identity of the recipient is not revealed by the surgical team, the likely media coverage will reveal their identity.

There is little doubt that face transplants will happen in the not too distant future. Once again, health psychologists are well placed to contribute to the process. This will include preparation for surgery – in particular assisting potential recipients to assimilate complex and detailed risk/benefit information; supporting decision making; contributing to realistic expectations about outcome, and providing ongoing support once the procedure has been completed (see Clarke and Butler 2004).

The impact of new appearance-enhancing procedures on society should not be underestimated. The publicity surrounding face transplantation may promote unrealistic expectations of the benefits, and is likely to further fuel the notion that a good quality of life cannot be achieved by people with an appearance that is visibly different. Acceptance of diversity in appearance may further decrease, and pressures on those with visible differences to seek treatment will increase. As Grealy (1994) said: '[others are] always telling her about the wonderful things surgeons can do nowadays'.

At this point in time, the dilemmas outlined above clearly raise more questions than there are answers. These represent just some of the fascinating issues that will continue to be a source of interest, concern and opportunities for health psychologists in the future and we look forward with anticipation to the discussions and work ahead.

**Further reading**

Clarke, A. and Butler, P.E.M. (2004) Face transplantation: psychological assessment and preparation for surgery. *Psychology, Health and Medicine*, 9: 315–26.

Kemp, S., Bruce, V. and Linney, A. (2004) *Future Face: Image, Identity and Innovation*. London: Profile Books.

Morris, P., Bradley, A., Doyal, L., Earley, M., Hagan, P., Milling, M. and Rumsey, N. (2004) Facial transplantation: is the time right?. *Transplantation*, 77: 329–38.

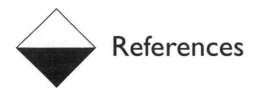

# References

Abel, T. (1952) Personality characteristics of the facially disfigured. *Transactions of the New York Academy of Sciences*, 4: 325–9.

Adachi, T., Kochi, S. and Yamaguchi, T. (2003) Characteristics of nonverbal behaviour in patients with cleft lip and palate during interpersonal communication. *Cleft Palate-Craniofacial Journal*, 40: 310–16.

Adams, G. and Crossman, S. (1978) *Physical Attractiveness: A Cultural Imperative*. Rosslyn Heights, NY: Libra.

Agar, N. (1998) Liberal eugenics, chapter 18, in H. Kuhse and P. Singer (eds) *Bioethics: An Anthology*. Oxford: Blackwell.

Altabe, M. and Thompson, J.K. (1996) Body image: a cognitive self-schema construct. *Cognitive Therapy and Research*, 20: 171–93.

Ambler, N., Rumsey, N., Harcourt, D., Khan, F., Cawthorn, S. and Barker, J. (1999) Specialist nurse counsellor interventions at the time of diagnosis of breast cancer: comparing 'advocacy' with a conventional approach. *Journal of Advanced Nursing*, 29: 445–53.

Andrews, B. (1998) Shame and childhood sexual abuse, in P. Gilbert and B. Andrews (eds) *Shame: Interpersonal Behavior, Psychopathology and Culture*, pp. 176–90. New York: Oxford University Press.

Appleyard, B. (1999) *Brave New Worlds: Genetics and the Human Experience*. London: HarperCollins.

Argyle, M. and McHenry, R. (1971) Do spectacles really affect judgments of intelligence? *British Journal of Social and Clinical Psychology*, 4: 27–9.

Armstrong, M.L. and Murphy, K.P. (1997) Tattooing: another adolescent risk behavior warranting health education. *Applied Nursing Research*, 10: 181–9.

Augustin, M., Zschocke, I., Peschen, M. and Vanscheidt, W. (1998) Psychosocial stress of patients with port wine stains and expectations of dye laser treatment. *Dermatology*, 197: 353–60.

Bacon, F. (1597) *The Essayes or Covnsels Civill and Morall of Francis Bacon*. Available at: http://darkwing.uoregon.edu/%7Erbear/bacon.html.

Baker, C. (1992) Factors associated with rehabilitation in head and neck cancer. *Cancer Nursing*, 15: 395–400.

Banister, E.M. (1999) Women's midlife experience of their changing bodies. *Qualitative Health Research*, 9: 520–37.

Barden, R.C., Ford, M.E., Jensen, A.G. and Salyer, K.E. (1989) Effects of craniofacial deformity in infancy on the quality of mother–infant interactions, *Child Development*, 60, 819–24.

Batchelor, D. (2001) Hair and cancer chemotherapy: consequences and nursing care – a literature study. *European Journal of Cancer Care*, 10: 147–63.

Bates, B. and Cleese, J. (2001) *The Human Face*, New York: DK Publishing.

Baumeister, R. (1997) Identity, self concept and self esteem: the self lost and found, in R. Hogan, J. Johnson and S. Briggs (eds) *Handbook of Personality Psychology*. New York: Academic Press.

Baumeister, R. and Leary, M.R. (1995) The need to belong: desire for interpersonal attachments as a fundamental human motivation. *Psychological Bulletin*, 117: 497–529.

Bayat, A., McGrouther, D.A. and Ferguson, M.W.J. (2003) Skin scarring. *BMJ*, 326: 88–92.

Beale, S., Lisper, H.O. and Palm, B. (1980) A psychological study of patients seeking augmentation mammaplasty. *The British Journal of Psychiatry*, 136: 133–8.

Beaune, L., Forrest, C.R. and Keith, T. (2004) Adolescents' perspectives on living and growing up with Treacher Collins Syndrome: a qualitative study, *Cleft Palate – Craniofacial Journal*, 41: 343–50.

Beebe, D.W., Hombeck, G.N., Schober, A., Lane, M. and Rosa, K. (1996) Is body focus restricted to self evaluation? Body focus in the evaluation of self and others. *International Journal of Eating Disorders*, 20: 415–22.

Ben-Tovim, D.I. and Walker, M.K. (1995) Body image, disfigurement and disability. *Journal of Psychosomatic Research*, 39: 283–91.

Bennett, P. (2004) Psychological interventions in patients with chronic illness, in A. Kaptein and J. Weinman (eds) *Health Psychology*. Oxford: BPS Blackwell.

Bennett, P. and Murphy, S. (1997) *Psychology and Health Promotion*. Buckingham: Open University Press.

Bernstein, N. (1976) *Emotional Care of the Facially Burned and Disfigured*. Boston: Little, Brown.

Berscheid, E. (1981) An overview of the psychological effects of physical attractiveness, in G. Lucker, K. Ribbens and J. McNamara (eds) *Psychological Aspects Official Form*. Ann Arbor: University of Michigan Press.

Berscheid, E. (1986) The question of the importance of physical attractiveness, in C. Herman, M. Zanna and E. Higgins (eds) *Physical Appearance, Stigma and Social Behavior*. Hillsdale, NJ: Lawrence Erlbaum.

Birdsall, C. and Weinberg, K. (2001) Adult patients looking at their burn injuries for the first time. *Journal of Burn Care and Rehabilitation*, 22: 360–4.

Bjelland, I., Dahl, A.A., Haug, T.T. and Neckelmann, D. (2002) The validity of the Hospital Anxiety and Depression Scale. An updated literature review. *Journal of Psychosomatic Research*, 2: 69–77.

Blakeney, P., Herndon, D.N., Desai, M.H., Beard, S. and Wales-Seale, P. (1988) Long-term psychosocial adjustment following burn injury. *Journal of Burn Care and Rehabilitation*, 9: 661–5.

Blakeney, P., Portman, S. and Rutan, R. (1990) Familial values as factors influencing long-term psychological adjustment of children after severe burn injury. *Journal of Burn Care and Rehabilitation*, 11: 472–5.

Blood, G.W. and Hyman, M. (1977) Children's perceptions of nasal resonance. *Journal of Speech and Hearing Discord*, 42: 446–8.

Bluman, L.G., Borstelmann, N.A., Rimer, B.K., Iglehart, J.D. and Winer, E.P. (2001) Knowledge, satisfaction and perceived cancer risk among women diagnosed with ductal carcinoma in situ. *Journal of Women's Health and Gender Based Medicine*, 10: 589–98.

Bond, M.J. and McDowell, A.J. (2001) An adolescent conception of body image and weight loss behaviours. *Journal of Applied Health Psychology*, 3: 8–15.

Bottomley, A. (1997) To randomize or not to randomize: methodological pitfalls of the RCT design in psychosocial intervention studies. *European Journal of Cancer Care*, 6: 222–30.

Bowling, A. (1997) *Research Methods in Health*. Buckingham: Open University Press.

Bradbury, E. (1993) Psychological approaches to children and adolescents with disfigurement: a review of the literature. *ACPP Review and Newsletter*, 15: 1–6.

Bradbury, E. (1997) Understanding the problems, in R. Lansdown, N. Rumsey, E. Bradbury, T. Carr and J. Partridge (eds) *Visibly Different: Coping with Disfigurement*. Oxford: Butterworth-Heinemann.

Bradbury, E. and Hewison, J. (1994) Early parental adjustment to visible congenital disfigurements. *Child: Care, Health and Development*, 20: 251–66.

Bradbury, E. and Middleton, J. (1997) Patient involvement in decision making about treatment, in R. Lansdown, N. Rumsey, E. Bradbury, T. Carr and J. Partridge (eds) *Visibly Different: Coping with Disfigurement*. Oxford: Butterworth-Heinemann.

Brandberg, Y., Malm, M., Rutqvist, L.-E., Jonsson, E. and Blomqvist, L. (1999) A prospective randomised study (named SVEA) of three methods of delayed breast reconstruction. Study design, patients' preoperative problems and expectations. *Scandinavian Journal of Plastic and Reconstructive Hand Surgery*, 33: 209–16.

British Medical Association (BMA) (2000) *BMA Takes Part in Body Image Summit*. Available at: www.bma.org.uk.

Broder, H. (2001) Using psychological assessment and therapeutic strategies to enhance well-being. *Cleft Palate-Craniofacial Journal*, 38: 248–54.

Broomfield, D., Humphris, G.M., Fisher, S.E., Vaughan, D., Brown, J.S. and Lane, S. (1997) The orofacial cancer patient's support from the general practitioner, hospital teams, family and friends. *Journal Cancer Education*, 12: 229–32.

Brown, B., Roberts, J., Browne, G., Byrne, C., Love, B. and Streiner, D. (1988) Gender differences in variables associated with psychosocial adjustment to a burn injury. *Research in Nursing and Health*, 11: 23–30.

Brown, M., Koch, T. and Webb, C. (2000) Information needs of women with non-invasive breast cancer. *Journal of Clinical Nursing*, 9: 713–22.

Browne, G., Byrne, C., Browne, B., Pennock, M., Streiner, D., Roberts, R., Eyles, P., Truscott, D. and Dabbs, R. (1985) Psychosocial adjustment of burns survivors. *Burns*, 12: 28–35.

Bruce, V. and Young, A. (1998) *In the Eye of the Beholder: The Science of Face Perception*. Oxford: Oxford University Press.

Bull, R. (1979) The psychological significance of facial deformity, in M. Cook and G. Wilson (eds) *Love and Attraction*. Oxford: Pergamon.

Bull, R. and Rumsey, N. (1988) *The Social Psychology of Facial Appearance*. London: Springer-Verlag.

Bull, R. and Stevens, J. (1981) The effects of facial disfigurement on helping behaviour. *Italian Journal of Psychology*, 8: 25–33.

Bull, R., Jenkins, M. and Stevens, J. (1983) Evaluation of politicians' faces. *Political Psychology*, 4: 713–16.

Burr, C. (1935) Personality and physiognomy, in *The Human Face: A Symposium*. Philadelphia: The Dental Cosmos.

Calman-Hine (1995) Policy framework for commissioning cancer services, Dept. of Health.

Cameron, L.D. and Nicholls, G. (1998) Expression of stressful experiences through writing: effects of a self-regulation manipulation for pessimists and optimists. *Health Psychology*, 17: 84–92.

Carmel, S., Shani, E. and Rosenberg, L. (1994) The role of age and an expanded health belief model in predicting skin cancer protective behaviour. *Health Education Research*, 9: 433–47.

Carr, A. (2004) *Positive Psychology: The Science of Happiness and Human Strengths*. Hove: Brunner-Routledge.

Carr, A.T., Harris, D.L. and James, C. (2000) The Derriford Appearance Scale: a new scale to measure individual responses to living with problems of appearance. *British Journal of Health Psychology*, 5: 201–15.

Carr, T., Moss, T. and Harris, D. (2005) The DAS24: A short form of the Derriford Appearance Scale (DAS59) to measure individual responses to living with problems of appearance. *British Journal of Health Psychology*, 10: 285–98.

Cash, T.F. (1992) The psychological effects of androgenetic alopecia in men. *Journal of the American Academy of Dermatology*, 26: 926–31.

Cash, T.F. (1996) The treatment of body image disturbances, in J.K. Thompson (ed.) *Body Image, Eating Disorders, and Obesity: An Integrative Guide for Assessment and Treatment*, pp. 83–107. Washington, DC: APA.

Cash, T.F. (1997) *The Body Image Workbook: An 8-step Programme for Learning to Like your Looks*. Oakland: New Harbinger Publications.

Cash, T.F. (2002a) Beyond traits: assessing body image states, in T.F. Cash and T. Pruzinsky (eds) *Body Image: A Handbook of Theory, Research and Clinical Practice*, London: The Guilford Press.

Cash, T.F. (2002b) Cognitive-behavioral perspectives on body image, in T.F. Cash and T. Pruzinsky (eds) *Body Image: A Handbook of Theory, Research and Clinical Practice*. London: The Guilford Press.

Cash, T.F. (2004) Body image: past, present and future. *Body Image*, 1: 1–5.

Cash, T. and Derlega, V. (1978) The matching hypothesis: physical attractiveness among same-sexed friends. *Personality and Social Psychology Bulletin*, 4: 240–3.

Cash, T.F. and Labarge, A.S. (1996) Development of the Appearance Schemas Inventory: a new cognitive body-image assessment. *Cognitive Therapy and Research*, 20: 37–50.

Cash, T.F. and Lavallee, D.M. (1997) Cognitive-behavioral body-image therapy: further evidence of the efficacy of a self-directed program. *Journal of Rational-Emotive and Cognitive-Behaviour Therapy*, 15: 281–94.

Cash, T. and Pruzinsky, T. (1990) *Body Image: Development, Deviance and Change*, London: The Guilford Press.

Cash, T.F. and Pruzinsky, T. (2002) *Body Image: A Handbook of Theory, Research and Clinical Practice*, London: The Guilford Press.

Cash, T.F. and Pruzinsky, T. (2002) Future challenges for body image theory, research and clinical practice, in T.F. Cash and T. Pruzinsky (eds) *Body Image: A Handbook of Theory, Research and Clinical Practice*, pp. 509–16. London: The Guilford Press.

Cash, T.F. and Strachan, M.D. (2002) Cognitive-behavioral approaches to changing body image, in T.F. Cash and T. Pruzinsky, T. (eds) *Body Image: A Handbook of Theory, Research and Clinical Practice*. London: The Guilford Press.

Cash, T.F., Melnyk, S.E. and Hrabosky, J.I. (2004) The assessment of body image investment: an extensive revision of the Appearance Schemas Inventory. *International Journal of Eating Disorders*, 35: 305–16.

Cash, T.F., Winstead, B.A. and Janda, L.H. (1986) The great American shape-up. *Psychology Today*, 20: 30–7.

Cash, T.F., Fleming, E.C., Alindogan, J., Steadman, L. and Whitehead, A. (2002) Beyond body image as a trait: the development and validation of the Body Images States Scale. *Eating Disorders: The Journal of Treatment and Prevention*, 10: 103–13.

Castle, C.M., Skinner, T.C. and Hampson, S.E. (1999) Young women and suntanning: an evaluation of a health education leaflet. *Psychology and Health*, 14: 517–27.

Chaikin, A., Gillen, B., Derlega, V., Heinen, J. and Wilson, M. (1978) Students' reactions to teachers' physical attractiveness and nonverbal behavior: two explanatory studies. *Psychology in the Schools*, 15: 588–95.

Charlton, R., Rumsey, N., Partridge, J., Barlow, J. and Saul, K. (2003) Editorial – Disfigurement – neglected in primary care? *British Journal of Primary Care*, 53: 6–8.

Chaudhary, V. (1996) The state we're in. *The Guardian*, 11 June.

Ching, S., Thomas, A., McCabe, R.E. and Antony, M.M. (2002) Measuring outcomes in aesthetic surgery: a comprehensive review of the literature. *Plastic and Reconstructive Surgery*, 111: 469–80.

Clarke, A. (1999) Psychosocial aspects of facial disfigurement: problems, management and the role of a lay-led organization. *Psychology, Health and Medicine*, 4: 128–41.

Clarke, A. (2001) Managing the psychological aspects of altered appearance: the development of an information resource for people with disfiguring conditions. *Patient Education and Counseling*, 43: 305–9.

Clarke, A. and Butler, P.E.M. (2004) Face transplantation: psychological assessment and preparation for surgery. *Psychology, Health and Medicine*, 9: 315–26.

Clarke, A. and Cooper, C. (2001) Psychological rehabilitation after disfiguring injury or disease: investigating the training needs of specialist nurses. *Journal of Advanced Nursing*, 34: 18–26.

Clarke, A. and Kish, V. (1998) *Exploring Faces Through Fiction*. London: Changing Faces.

Clarke, A., Rumsey, N., Collin, J.R.O. and Wyn-Williams, M. (2003) Psychosocial distress associated with disfiguring eye conditions. *Eye*, 17: 35–40.

Clifford, E. (1973) Psychological aspects of orofacial anomalies: speculations in search of data, in *Orofacial Anomalies: Clinical and Research Implications*. Rockville, MD: American Speech and Hearing Association.

Cline, T., Proto, A., Raval, P. and Di Paolo, T. (1998) The effects of brief exposure and of classroom teaching on attitudes children express towards facial disfigurement in peers. *Educational Research*, 40: 55–68.

Clinical Standards Advisory Group (CSAG) (1998) *Cleft Lip and/or Palate*. London: HMSO.

Cochrane, V.M. and Slade, P. (1999) Appraisal and coping in adults with cleft lip: associations with well-being and social anxiety. *British Journal of Medical Psychology*, 72: 485–503.

Concar, D. (2004) The boldest cut. *New Scientist*, 29 May.

Cook, S. (1939) The judgment of intelligence from photographs. *Journal of Abnormal and Social Psychology*, 23: 33–9.

Cooper, C. (2000) Face on: discovering resilience to disfigurement. *The New Therapist*, Vol. 7, No. 3, pp. 31–3.

Cooper, M. (1997) Do interpretive biases maintain eating disorders? *Behaviour Research and Therapy*, 35: 363–5.

Cooper, J.M. and Clarke, A. (1999) *Expert Patients: Who Are They? Lay-led Self-management Programmes: An Additional Resource in the Management of Chronic Illness*, for The Long-Term Medical Conditions Alliance (LMCA). Available at: www.lmca.org.uk/docs/article.htm.

Cooper, R. and Burnside, I. (1996) Three years of an adult burns support group: an analysis. *Burns*, 22: 65–8.

Coopersmith, S. (1967) *Antecedents of Self Esteem*. London: Freeman.

Cotterill, J. and Cunliffe, W. (1997) Suicide in dermatological patients. *British Journal of Dermatology*, 137: 246–50.

Coughlan, G. and Clarke, A. (2002) Shame and burns, in P. Gilbert and J. Miles (eds) *Body Shame*. Hove: Brunner-Routledge.

Coyne, J.C. and Gottlieb, B.H. (1996) The mismeasure of coping by checklist. *Journal of Personality*, 64: 961–91.

Crittenden, P. and Ainsworth, M. (1989) Child maltreatment and attachment theory, in D. Cicchetti and V. Carlson *Child Maltreatment*. New York: Cambridge University Press.

Crozier, W.R. (2001) *Understanding Shyness: Psychological Perspectives*. Basingstoke: Palgrave Macmillan.

Crozier, W.R. and Dimmock, P.S. (1999) Name-calling and nicknames in a sample of primary school children. *British Journal of Educational Psychology*, 69: 505–16.

Cusumano, D. and Thompson, J. (2001) Media influence and body image in 8–11 year old boys and girls: a preliminary report on the Multidimensional Media Influence Scale, *International Journal of Eating Disorders*, 29: 37–44.

Davalbhakta, A. and Hall, P.N. (2000) The impact of antenatal diagnosis on the effectiveness and timing of counselling for cleft lip and palate. *British Journal of Plastic Surgery*, 53: 298–301.

Davis, K. (1995) *Reshaping the Female Body: The Dilemma of Cosmetic Surgery*. New York: Routledge.

Dean, C., Chetty, U. and Forrest, A. (1983) Effects of immediate breast reconstruction on psychosocial morbidity after mastectomy. *The Lancet*: 459–62.

Deber, R.B., Kraetschmer, N. and Irvine, J. (1996) What role do patients wish to play in treatment decision making? *Archives of Internal Medicine*, 156: 1414–20.

Dee, J. (2001) *The Complete Guide to Chinese Face Reading*. Cullompton: D & S Books.

Demarest, J. and Allen, R. (2000) Body image: gender, ethnic and age differences. *Journal of Social Psychology*, 140: 465–72.

De Morgan, S., Redman, S., White, K.J., Cakir, B. and Boyages, J. (2002) 'Well, have I got cancer or haven't I?' The psycho-social issues for women diagnosed with ductal carcinoma in situ. *Health Expectations*, 5: 310–18.

Department of Health *Hospital Episode Statistics 2000–2001*. London: Department of Health.

Department of Health (2004) *Choosing Health: Making Healthy Choices Easier – White Paper*. London: Department of Health.

Dew, M., Dunbar-Jacob, J., Switzer, G., DiMartini, A., Stilley, C. and Kormos, R. (2001) Adherence to the medical regimen in transplantation, in J. Rodrigue (ed.) *Biopsychosocial Perspective on Transplantation*. New York: Kluwer Academic.

Dion, K. (1973) Young children's stereotyping of facial attractiveness. *Developmental Psychology*, 9: 183–8.

Dion, K., Berscheid, E. and Walster, E. (1972) What is beautiful is good. *Journal of Personality and Social Psychology*, 24: 285–90.

Dittmar, H., Lloyd, B., Dugan, S., Halliwell, E., Cramer, H. and Jacobs, N. (2001) The 'body beautiful': English adolescents' images of ideal bodies. *Sex Roles*, 42: 887–915.

Donaldson, C. (1996) A study of male body image and the effects of the media. Unpublished BSc dissertation, Manchester Metropolitan University.

Dropkin, M.J. (1989) Coping with disfigurement and dysfunction after head and neck cancer surgery: a conceptual framework. *Seminars in Oncology Nursing*, 5: 213–19.

Dropkin, M.J. (1999) Body image and quality of life after head and neck cancer surgery. *Cancer Practice*, 7: 309–13.

Dropkin, M.J. (2001) Anxiety, coping strategies and coping behaviours in patients undergoing head and neck cancer surgery. *Cancer Nursing*, 24: 143–8.

Duncan, M.J., Al-Nakeeb, Y. and Nevill, A.M. (2004) Body esteem and body fat in British school children from different ethnic groups. *Body Image*, 1: 311–15.

Eagly, A.H., Ashmore, R.D., Makhijani, M.G. and Longo, L.C. (1991) What is beautiful is good, but . . .: a meta analytic review of research on the physical attractiveness stereotype. *Psychological Bulletin*, 110: 109–28.

Eiser, C. (1998) Practitioner review: long-term consequences of childhood cancer. *Journal of Child Psychology and Psychiatry*, 39: 621–33.

Eiserman, W. (2001) Unique outcomes and positive contributions associated with facial difference: expanding research and practice. *Cleft Palate Craniofacial Journal*, 3: 236–44.

Elmendorf, E.N., D'Antonio, L.L. and Hardesty, R.A. (1993) Assessment of the patient with cleft lip and palate. *Clinics in Plastic Surgery*, 20: 607–21.

Emerson, M. and Rumsey, N. (2004) Psychosocial audit off cleft-affected patients. Unpublished conference paper at annual conference of the Craniofacial Society of Great Britain and Ireland, Bath.

Endriga, M.C. and Kapp-Simon, K.A. (1999) Psychological issues in craniofacial care: state of the art. *Cleft Palate Craniofacial Journal*, 36: 3–9.

Engel, G.L. (1977) The need for a new model: a challenge for biomedicine. *Science*, 196: 129–36.

Etcoff, N. (1999) *Survival of the Prettiest: The Science of Beauty*. London: Little, Brown and Company.

Fabian, L.J. and Thompson, J.K. (1989) Body image and eating disturbance in young females. *International Journal of Eating Disorders*, 8: 63–74.

Fallowfield, L. and Clarke, A. (1991) *Breast Cancer*. London: Routledge.

Farrimond, J. and Morris, M. (2004) Knowing or not knowing before birth: parents' experiences of having a baby with a cleft malformation. Paper presented at the

British Psychological Society Division of Health Psychology annual conference, Edinburgh, September 2004.

Feingold, A. (1988) Matching for attractiveness in romantic partners and same sex friends. A meta analysis and theoretical critique. *Psychology Bulletin*, 104: 226–35.

Feingold, A. (1992) Good looking people are not what we think. *Psychological Bulletin*, 111: 304–41.

Feingold, A. and Mazzella, R. (1998) Gender differences in body image are increasing. *Psychological Science*, 9: 190–5.

Festinger, L. (1954) A theory of social comparison processes. *Human Relations*, 7: 117–40.

Field, T. and Vega-Lahr, N. (1984) Early interactions between infants with craniofacial abnormalities and their mothers. *Infant Behavior and Development*, 7: 527–30.

Fisher, S. and Cleveland, B. (1958) *Body Image and Personality*. New York: Dover Publications.

Fortune, D.G., Richards, H.L., Griffiths, C.E.M. and Main, C.J. (2005) Adversarial growth in patients undergoing treatment for psoriasis: a prospective study of the ability of patients to construe benefits from negative events. *Psychology, Health and Medicine*, 10: 44–56.

Fortune, D.G., Richards, H.L., Main, C.J. and Griffiths, C.E.M. (2000) Pathological worrying, illness perceptions and disease severity in patients with psoriasis. *British Journal of Health Psychology*, 5: 71–82.

Fortune, D.G., Richards, H.L, Main, C.J., O'Sullivan, T.M. and Griffiths, C.E.M. (1998) Developing clinical psychology services in an out-patient dermatology clinic: what factors are associated with non-uptake of the service? *Clinical Psychology Forum*, 115: 34–7.

Frances, J. (2000) Providing effective support in school when a child has a disfigurement. *Support for Learning*, 15: 177–82.

Freedman, R. (1986) *Beauty Bound*. Lexington, MA: Heath.

Frith, H. and Gleeson, K. (2004) Clothing and embodiment: men managing body image and appearance. *Psychology of Men and Masculinity*, 5: 40–8.

Frith, H. and Gleeson, K. (in press) Deconstructing body image. *Journal of Health Psychology*.

Frost, L. (2003) Doing bodies differently? Gender, youth, appearance and damage. *Journal of Youth Studies*, 6: 53–70.

Frost, M.H., Schaid, D.J., Sellars, T.A. et al. (2000) Long-term satisfaction and psychological and social function following bilateral prophylactic mastectomy. *JAMA*, 284: 319–24.

Frost, P. (1994) Preference for darker faces in photographs at different phases of the menstrual cycle: preliminary assessment of evidence for a hormonal relationship. *Perceptual Motor Skills*, 79: 507–14.

Gallagher, P. and MacLachlan, M. (2000) Positive meaning in amputation and thoughts about amputated limb. *Prosthetics and Orthotic International*, 24: 196–204.

Galton, F. (1883) *Inquiries into Human Faculty and Its Development*. London: Macmillan.

Gamba, A., Romano, M., Grosso, I.M., Tamburini, M., Cantu, G., Molinari, R. and Ventafridda, V. (1992) Psychosocial adjustment of patients surgically treated for head and neck cancer. *Head and Neck*, 14: 218–23.

Garner, D.M. (1997) The 1997 body image survey results. *Psychology Today*, 30: 30–44, 75–80, 84.

Gibbons, F.X. (1999) Social comparison as a mediator of response shift. *Social Science and Medicine*, 48: 1517–30.

Gilbert, P. (1997) The evolution of social attractiveness and its role in shame, humiliation, guilt and therapy. *British Journal of Medical Psychology*, 70: 19–22.

Gilbert, P. (2002) Body shame: a biopsychosocial conceptualization and overview, with treatment implications, in P. Gilbert and J. Miles (eds) *Body Shame: Conceptualisation, Research and Treatment*. Hove: Brunner-Routledge.

Gilbert, S. and Miles, J. (eds) (2002) *Body Shame: Conceptualisation, Research and Treatment*. Hove: Brunner-Routledge.

Gilbert, S. and Thompson, J. (2002) Body shame in childhood and adolescence, in P. Gilbert and J. Miles (eds) *Body Shame: Conceptualisation, Research and Treatment*. Hove: Brunner-Routledge.

Ginsberg, I. and Link, B. (1989) Feelings of stigmatization in patients with psoriasis. *Journal of the American Academy of Dermatology*, 20: 53–63.

Gittings, J. (2001) The unwanted: China's abandoned children. August 7th, 2001. *The Guardian*.

Goffman, E. (1963) *Stigma: Notes on the Management of Spoiled Identity*. Englewood Cliffs, NJ: Prentice-Hall.

Grant, P. (1996) If you could change your breasts . . . *Self*, 186–9, 210–11.

Grealy, L. (1994) *In the Mind's Eye: An Autobiography of a Face*. London: Arrow.

Green, J.D. and Sedikides, C. (2001) When do self-schemas shape social perception? The role of descriptive ambiguity. *Motivation and Emotion*, 25: 67–83.

Groesz, L.M., Levine, M.P. and Murnen, S.K. (2002) The effect of experimental presentation of thin media images on body satisfaction: a meta-analytic review. *International Journal of Eating Disorders*, 31: 1–16.

Grogan, S. (1999) *Body Image: Understanding Body Dissatisfaction in Men, Women and Children*. London: Routledge.

Haig-Ferguson, A. (2003) How do blind people construct their concept of body image? Unpublished thesis, University of Bath.

Haiken, E. (2000) The making of the modern face: cosmetic surgery. *Social Research*, 67: 82.

Hall, A. and Fallowfield, L. (1989) Psychological outcome of treatment for early breast cancer: a review. *Stress and Medicine*, 5: 167–75.

Hall, C. (1995) Asian eyes: Body image and eating disorders of Asian and Asian American women. *Eating Disorders: The Journal of Treatment and Prevention*, 3: 8–19.

Halliwell, E. and Dittmar, H. (2003) A qualitative investigation of women's and men's body image concerns and their attitudes towards aging. *Sex Roles*, 49: 675–84.

Halliwell, E. and Dittmar, H. (2004) Does size matter? The impact of model's body size on women's body-focused anxiety and advertising effectiveness. *Journal of Social and Clinical Psychology*, 23: 104–22.

Hamilton-West, K. and Bridle, C. (2004) Effects of written emotional disclosure following residential fire: triple blind randomized controlled trial. Paper presented at the British Psychological Society Division of Health Psychology Annual Conference, Edinburgh, September 2004.

Hanna, K.M. and Jacobs, P. (1993) The use of photography to explore the meaning of health among adolescents with cancer. *Issues in Comprehensive Pediatric Nursing*, 16: 155–64.

Hansen, K., Kreiter, C.D., Rosenbaum, M., Whitaker, D.C. and Arpey, C.J. (2003) Long-term psychological impact and perceived efficacy of pulsed-dye laser therapy for patients with port wine stains. *Dermatological Surgery*, 29: 49–55.

Harcourt, D. and Griffiths, C. (2003) Women's experiences of ductal carcinoma in situ (DCIS). Paper presented at the British Psychological Society Division of Health Psychology Annual Conference, Stafford, September 2003.

Harcourt, D. and Rumsey, N. (2001) Psychological aspects of breast reconstruction: a review of the literature. *Journal of Advanced Nursing*, 35: 477–87.

Harcourt, D. and Rumsey, N. (2004) Mastectomy patients' decision-making for or against immediate breast reconstruction. *Psycho-Oncology*, 13: 106–15.

Harcourt, D., Rumsey, N., Ambler, N., Cawthorn, S.J., Reid, C., Maddox, P., Kenealy, J., Rainsbury, R. and Umpleby, H. (2003) The psychological impact of mastectomy with or without immediate breast reconstruction: a prospective, multi-centred study. *Plastic and Reconstructive Surgery*, 111: 1060–8.

Hari, J. (2003) Plastic surgery won't make you beautiful. *The Independent*, 26 November.

Harris, D. (1997) Types, causes and physical treatment, in R. Lansdown, N. Rumsey, E. Bradbury, T. Carr and J. Partridge (eds) *Visibly Different: Coping with Disfigurement*. Oxford: Butterworth-Heinemann.

Harris, D. and Carr, A. (2001) Prevalence of concern about physical appearance in the general population. *British Journal of Plastic Surgery*, 54: 223–6.

Harter, S. (1999) *The Construction of Self: A Developmental Perspective*. New York: The Guilford Press.

Haste, H. (2004) *My Body, My Self: Young People's Values and Motives About Healthy Living*. London: Nestlé Social Research Programme.

Hatcher, M. and Fallowfield, L. (2003) A qualitative study looking at the psycho-social implications of bilateral prophylactic mastectomy, *Breast*, 12: 1–9.

Hatcher, M.B., Fallowfield, L. and A'Hern, R. (2001) The psychosocial impact of bilateral prophylactic mastectomy: prospective study using questionnaires and semi-structured interviews. *BMJ*, 322: 76–9.

Hatfield, E. and Sprecher, S. (1986) *Mirror, Mirror . . . The Importance of Looks on Everyday Life*. New York: SUNY Press.

Hearst, D. and Middleton, J. (1997) Psychological intervention and models of current working practice, in R. Lansdown, N. Rumsey, E. Bradbury, T. Carr and J. Partridge (eds) *Visibly Different: Coping with Disfigurement*. Oxford: Butterworth-Heinemann.

Heason, S.L. (2003) The development of a model of disfigurement: the process of living with vitiligo. Unpublished PhD thesis, University of Sheffield.

Heatherton, T.F., Mahamedi, F., Striepe, M., Field, A.E. and Keel, P. (1997) A 10-year longitudinal study of body weight, dieting and eating disorder symptoms. *Journal of Abnormal Psychology*, 106: 117–25.

Heinberg, L.H. and Thompson, J.K. (1995) Body image and televised images of thinness and attractiveness: a controlled laboratory investigation. *Journal of Social and Clinical Psychology*, 14: 325–38.

Heinrichs, N. and Hoffmann, S.G. (2001) Information processing in social phobia: a critical review. *Clinical Psychology Review*, 21: 751–70.

Herskind, A.M., Christensen, K., Juel, K. and Fogh-Anderson, P. (1993) Cleft lip: A risk factor for suicide. Paper presented at the 7th International Congress on cleft palate and related craniofacial anomalies, Australia.

Higgins, E.T. and Brendl, C.M. (1995) Accessibility and applicability: some 'activation rules' influencing judgement. *Journal of Experimental Social Psychology*, 31: 218–43.

Hill, L. and Kennedy, P. (2002) The role of coping strategies in mediating subjective disability in people with psoriasis. *Psychology, Health and Medicine*, 7: 261–9.

Holmes, S. and Hatch, C. (1938) Personal appearance as related to scholastic records and marriage selection in college women. *Human Biology*, 10: 65–76.

Holsen, I., Kraft, P. and Roysamb, E. (2001) The relationship between body image and depressed mood in adolescence: a 5-year longitudinal panel study. *Journal of Health Psychology*, 6: 613–27.

Hopwood, P. and Maguire, G.P. (1988) Body image problems in cancer patients. *British Journal of Psychiatry*, 153: 47–50.

Hopwood, P., Fletcher, I., Lee, A. and Al Ghazal, S. (2001) A body image scale for use with cancer patients. *European Journal of Cancer*, 37: 189–97.

Hopwood, P., Lee, A., Shenton, A., Baildam, A., Brain, A., Lalloo, F., Evans, G. and Howell, A. (2000) Clinical follow-up after bilateral risk reducing ('prophylactic') mastectomy: mental health and body image issues. *Psycho-Oncology*, 9: 462–72.

Horlock, N., Cole, R.P. and Rossi, A.R. (1999) The selection of patients for breast reduction: should health commissions have a say? *British Journal of Plastic Surgery*, 52: 118–21.

Houghton, S., Durkin, K. and Carroll, A. (1995) Children's and adolescents' awareness of the physical and mental health risks associated with tattooing: a focus group study. *Adolescence*, 30: 971–88.

Houston, V. and Bull, R. (1994) Do people avoid sitting next to someone who is facially disfigured? *European Journal of Social Psychology*, 24: 279–84.

Hughes, M. (1998) *The Social Consequences of Facial Disfigurement*. Aldershot: Ashgate Publishing.

Humphreys, P. and Paxton, S.J. (2004) Impact of exposure to idealized male images on adolescent boys' body image. *Body Image*, 1: 253–66.

Hutton, J.M. and Williams, M. (2001) Assessment of psychological issues and needs in the specialties of a large teaching hospital. *Psychology, Health and Medicine*, 6: 313–19.

Iliffee, A. (1960) A study of preferences in feminine beauty. *British Journal of Psychology*, 51: 267–73.

Jackman, L.P., Williamson, D.A., Netemeyer, R.G. and Anderson, D.A. (1995) Do weight preoccupied women misinterpret ambiguous stimuli related to body size? *Cognitive Therapy and Research*, 19: 341–55.

Joachim, G. and Acorn, S. (2003) Life with a rare chronic disease: the scleroderma experience. *Journal of Advanced Nursing*, 42: 598–606.

Johnson, S., Burrows, A. and Williamson, I. (2004) 'Does my bump look big in this?' The meaning of bodily changes for first-time mothers-to-be. *Journal of Health Psychology*, 9: 361–74.

Johnston, O., Reilly, J. and Kremer, J. (2004) Women's experiences of appearance concern and body control across the lifespan: challenging accepted wisdom. *Journal of Health Psychology*, 9: 397–410.

Jones, D. and Hill, K. (1993) Criteria of physical attractiveness in five populations. *Human Nature*, 4: 271–96.

Jones, E.E., Farina, A., Hastorf, A.H., Markus, H., Miller, D.T., Scott, R.A. and de S. French, R. (1984) *Social Stigma: The Psychology of Marked Relationships.* New York: W. H. Freeman and Company.

Jones, J.L. and Leary, M.R. (1994) Effects of appearance-based admonitions against sun-exposure on tanning intentions in young adults. *Health Psychology*, 13: 86–90.

Jowett, S. and Ryan, T. (1985) Skin disease and handicap: an analysis of the impact of skin conditions. *Social Science and Medicine*, 20: 425–9.

Kapp-Simon, K.A. (1995) Psychological interventions for the adolescent with cleft lip and palate. *Cleft Palate Craniofacial Journal*, 32: 104–8.

Kapp-Simon, K.A. and Dawson, P. (1998) Behavior adjustment and competence of children with craniofacial conditions. Paper presented at the Annual Meeting of the American Cleft-Palate Craniofacial Association, Baltimore, April 1998.

Kapp-Simon, K.A. and McGuire, D. (1997) Observed social interaction patterns in adolescents with and without craniofacial conditions. *Cleft Palate Craniofacial Journal*, 34: 380–4.

Kapp-Simon, K.A., Simon, D.J. and Kristovitch, S. (1992) Self-perception, social skill, adjustment and inhibition in young adolescents with craniofacial anomalies. *Cleft Palate Craniofacial Journal*, 29: 352–7.

Kearney-Cooke, A. (2002) Familial influences on body image development, in T.F. Cash and T. Pruzinsky (eds) *Body Image: A Handbook of Theory, Research and Clinical Practice.* New York: The Guilford Press.

Kellett, S. (2002) Shame-fused acne: a biopsychosocial conceptualization and treatment rationale, in P. Gilbert and J. Miles (eds) *Body Shame.* Hove: Brunner-Routledge.

Kemp, S., Bruce, V. and Linney, A. (2004) *Future Face: Image, Identity, Innovation.* London: Profile Books.

Kennedy, I. (1988) The technological imperative and its application in health care, in *Treat Me Right: Essays in Medicine, Law and Ethics.* Oxford: Clarendon Press.

Kent, G. (1999) Correlates of perceived stigma in vitiligo. *Psychology and Health*, 14: 241–52.

Kent, G. (2000) Understanding the experiences of people with disfigurements: an integration of four models of social and psychological functioning. *Psychology, Health and Medicine*, 5: 117–29.

Kent, G. (2002) Testing a model of disfigurement: effects of a skin camouflage service on well-being and appearance anxiety. *Psychology and Health*, 17: 377–86.

Kent, G. and Keahone, S. (2001) Social anxiety and disfigurement: the moderating effects of fear of negative evaluation and past experience. *British Journal of Clinical Psychology*, 40: 23–34.

Kent, G. and Thompson, A.R. (2002) The development and maintenance of shame in disfigurement: Implications for treatment, in P. Gilbert and J. Miles (eds) *Body Shame.* Hove: Brunner-Routledge.

King, M.T., Kenny, P., Shiell, A., Hall, J. and Boyages, J. (2000) Quality of life three months and one year after first treatment for early-stage breast cancer: influence of treatment and patient characteristics. *Quality of Life Research*, 9: 789–800.

Kish, V. and Lansdown, R. (2000) Meeting the psychosocial impact of facial disfigurement: developing a clinical service for children and families. *Clinical Child Psychology and Psychiatry*, 5: 497–511.

Klassen, A., Fitzpatrick, R., Jenkinson, C. and Goodacre, T. (1996) Patients' health-related quality of life before and after aesthetic surgery. *British Journal of Plastic Surgery*, 49: 433–8.

Kleck, R. and Strenta, A. (1980) Perceptions of the impact of negatively valued physical characteristics on social interaction. *Journal of Personality and Social Psychology*, 39: 861–73.

Kleinke, C. (1974) *First Impressions: The Psychology of Encountering Others*. Englewood Cliffs, NJ: Prentice Hall.

Kleve, L. and Robinson, E. (1999) A survey of psychological need amongst adult burn-injured patients. *Burns*, 25: 575–9.

Kleve, L., Rumsey, N., Wyn-Williams, M. and White, P. (2002) The effectiveness of cognitive-behavioural interventions provided at Outlook: a disfigurement support unit. *Journal of Evaluation in Clinical Practice*, 8: 387–95.

Kligman, A. (1989) Psychological aspects of skin disorders in the elderly. *Cutis*, 43: 498–501.

Koo, J. (1995) The psychosocial impact of acne: patients' perceptions. *Journal of the American Academy of Dermatology*, 32: 26–30.

Krueckeberg, S., Kapp-Simon, K. and Ribordy, S. (1993) Social skills of preschoolers with and without craniofacial anomalies. *Cleft Palate Craniofacial Journal*, 30(5): 475–81.

Lakoff, R. and Scherr, R. (1984) *Face Value: The Politics of Beauty*. Boston: Routledge and Kegan Paul.

Lander, E. (1992) Winding your way through DNA. Symposium, University of California, San Francisco. Available at: www.accessexcellence.org/RC/CC/lander.html.

Lanigan, S. and Cotterill, J. (1989) Psychological disabilities amongst patients with port wine stains. *British Journal of Dermatology*, 121: 451–63.

Langer, E., Fiske, S., Taylor, S. and Chanowitz, B. (1976) Stigma, staring and discomfort: a novel-stimulus hypothesis. *Journal of Experimental Social Psychology*, 12: 451–63.

Langlois, J. (1986) From the eye of the beholder to behavioral reality: development of social behaviors and social relations as a function of physical attractiveness, in C. Herman, M. Zanna and E. Higgins (eds) *Physical Appearance, Stigma, and Social Behavior*. Hillsdale, NJ: Lawrence Erlbaum.

Langlois, J.H., Kalakanis, L., Rubenstein, A.J., Larson, A., Hallam, M. and Smoot, M. (2000) Maxims or myths of beauty? A meta-analytic and theoretical review. *Psychological Bulletin*, 126: 390–423.

Lansdown, R. (1976) *The Psychological Management of Children with a Facial Deformity*. (Available from the author, The Hospital for Sick Children, Great Ormond Street, London, UK.)

Lansdown, R., Rumsey, N., Bradbury, E., Carr, T. and Partridge, J. (1997) *Visibly Different: Coping with Disfigurement*. Oxford: Butterworth-Heinemann.

Lavater, J.C. (1789) *Essays on Physiognomy*. London: Thomas Tegg.

Leary, M. (1990) Responses to social exclusion: social anxiety, jealousy, loneliness, depression and low self-esteem. *Journal of Social and Clinical Psychology*, 9: 221–9.

Leary, M., Rapp, S., Herbst, K., Exum, M. and Feldman, S. (1998) Interpersonal concerns and psychological difficulties of psoriasis patients: effects of disease severity and fear of negative evaluation. *Health Psychology*, 17: 1–7.

Leary, M.R., Tchividjian, L.R. and Kraxberger, B.E. (1994) Self-presentation can be hazardous to your health: impression management and health risk. *Health Psychology*, 13: 461–70.

Lee, C. and Owens, R.G. (2002) *The Psychology of Men's Health*. Buckingham: Open University Press.

Leventhal, H., Meyer, D. and Nerenz, D. (1980) The commonsense representations of illness danger, in S. Rachman (ed.) *Medical Psychology*, Vol. 11. New York: Pergamon.

Levine, R.M. (1999) Identity and illness: the effects of identity salience and frame of reference of illness and injury. *British Journal of Health Psychology*, 4: 63–80.

Levine, M.P. and Smolak, L. (1992) Toward a developmental model of the psychopathology of eating disorders: the example of early adolescence, in J.H. Crowther, S.E. Hobfoll, D.L. Tennenbaum and M.A.P. Stephens (eds) *The Eitiology of Bulimia Nervosa: The Individual and Family Context*, pp. 59–80. Washington, DC: Hemisphere.

Levine, M.P. and Smolak, L. (1996) Media as a context for the development of disordered eating, in L. Smolak and M.P. Levine (eds) *The Developmental Psychopathology of Eating Disorders: Implications for Research, Prevention and Treatment*, pp. 235–57. Mahwah, NJ: Lawrence Erlbaum.

Levine, M.P. and Smolak, L. (2002) Body image development in adolescence. In T. Cash and T. Pruzinsky (eds) *Body Image: A Handbook of Theory, Research and Clinical Practice*, pp. 74–82. London: The Guilford Press.

Linney, A. (2004) Perils of Perfection, in Secrets of the Face Supplement to New Scientist, 2nd October, 2004, 6–7.

Liossi, C. (2003) Appearance related concerns across the general and clinical populations. Unpublished thesis, City University, London.

Lockhart, J.S. (1999) Nurses' perceptions of head and neck oncology patients and surgery: severity of facial disfigurement and patient gender. *Head and Neck Nursing*, 17: 12–25.

Lorig, K., Sobel, D.S., Stewart, A.L. et al. (1999) Evidence suggesting that a chronic disease self-management programme can improve health status while reducing hospitalisation: a randomised trial. *Medical Care*, 1: 5–14.

Love, B., Bryne, C., Roberts, J., Browne, G. and Brown, B. et al. (1987) Adult psychosocial adjustment following childhood injury: the effect of disfigurement. *Journal of Burn Care Rehabilitation*, 8: 280–5.

Lovegrove, E. (2002) Adolescence: Appearance and anti-bullying strategies, Unpublished PhD thesis, University of the West of England, UK.

Lovegrove, E. and Rumsey, N. (2005) Ignoring it doesn't make it stop: adolescents, appearance and anti-bullying strategies. *Cleft Palate-Craniofacial Journal*, 42: 33–44.

Lucker, G., Graber, L. and Pietromonaco, P. (1981) The importance of dentofacial appearance in facial esthetics: a signal detection approach. *Basic and Applied Psychology*, 2: 261–74.

MacGregor, F.C. (1970) Social and psychological implications of dentofacial disfigurement. *Angle Orthodontics*, 40: 231–3.

MacGregor, F.C. (1974) *Transformation and Identity: The Face and Plastic Surgery*. New York: Quadrangle/New York Times Books.

MacGregor, F.C. (1979) *After Plastic Surgery: Adaptation and Adjustment*. New York: Praeger.

MacGregor, F.C. (1989) Social, psychological and cultural dimensions of cosmetic and reconstructive plastic surgery. *Aesthetic Plastic Surgery*, 13: 1–8.

MacGregor, F.C. (1990) Facial disfigurement: problems and management of social interaction and implications for mental health. *Aesthetic Plastic Surgery*, 14: 249–57.

MacGregor, F.C., Abel, T.M., Bryt, A., Laver, E. and Weissman, S. (1953) *Facial Deformities and Plastic Surgery*. Springfield, IL: Thomas.

MacLachlan, M. (2004) *Embodiment: Clinical, Critical and Cultural Perspectives on Health and Illness*. Maidenhead: Open University Press.

Maddern, L. and Emerson, M. (2002) Outcomes of a psychological intervention for children with different appearance. Paper presented to the Annual Scientific Meeting of the Craniofacial Society of Great Britain and Ireland, East Grinstead, April 2002.

Maddern, L. and Owen, T. (2004) The Outlook summer group: a social skills workshop for children with a different appearance who are transferring to secondary school. *Clinical Psychology*, 33: 25–9.

Malt, U. and Ugland, O. (1989) A long-term psychosocial follow-up study of burned adults. *Acta Psychiatr. Scand. Suppl*, 355: 94–102.

Marks, D.F., Murray, M., Evans, B. and Willig, C. (2000) *Health Psychology: Theory, Research and Practice*. London: SAGE Publications.

Markus, H. (1977) Self-schemata and processing information about the self. *Journal of Personality and Social Psychology*, 35: 63–78.

Martin, C.R. and Newell, R. (2004) Factor structure of the Hospital Anxiety and Depression Scale in individuals with facial disfigurement. *Psychology, Health and Medicine*, 9: 327–36.

Matthews, M., Cohen, M., Viglione, M. and Brown, A. (1998) Prenatal counseling for cleft lip and palate. *Plastic and Reconstructive Surgery*, 101: 1–5.

McArthur, L. (1982) Judging a book by its cover: a cognitive analysis of the relationship between physical appearance and stereotyping, in A. Hastorf and A. Isen (eds) *Cognitive Social Psychology*. New York: Elsevier.

McCabe, M.P. and Ricciardelli, L.A. (2003) A longitudinal study of body change strategies among adolescent males. *Journal of Youth and Adolescence*, 32: 105–13.

McGarvey, E.L., Baum, L.D., Pinkerton, R.C. and Rogers, L.M. (2001) Psychological sequelae and alopecia among women with cancer. *Cancer Practice*, 9: 283–9.

McGrouther, D.A. (1997) Facial disfigurement. *BMJ*, 314: 991.

Melynk, S.E., Cash, T.F. and Janda, L.H. (2004) Body image ups and downs: prediction of intra-individual level and variability of women's daily body image experiences. *Body Image*, 1: 225–35.

Meyers-Paal, R., Blakeney, P., Robert, R., Murphy. L., Chinkers, D., Meyer, W., Desai, M. and Hendon, D. (2000) Physical and psychologic rehabilitation outcomes or pediatric patients who suffer 80% or more TBSA, 70% or more 3rd degree burns. *Journal of Burn Care Rehabilitation*, 21: 43–9.

Meyerson, M.D. (2001) Resiliency and success in adults with moebius syndrome. *Cleft Palate Craniofacial Journal*, 38: 232–5.

Miles, J. (2002) Psoriasis: the role of shame on quality of life, in P. Gilbert and J. Miles (eds) *Body Shame*, pp. 119–34. Hove: Brunner-Routledge.

Mintz, L.B. and Betz, N.E. (1986) Sex differences in the nature, realism and correlates of body image. *Sex Roles*, 15: 185–95.

Morris, P., Bradley, A., Doyal, L., Earley, M., Milling, M. and Rumsey, N. (2004) Facial transplantation: is the time right? *Transplantation*, 77: 329–38.

Montepare, J.M. (1996) An assessment of adults' perceptions of their psychological, physical and social age. *Journal of Clinical Geropsychology*, 2: 117–28.

Moss, T. (1997) Individual variation in adjusting to visible differences, in R. Lansdown, N. Rumsey, E. Bradbury, T. Carr and J. Partridge (eds) *Visibly Different: Coping with Disfigurement*. Oxford: Butterworth-Heinemann.

Moss, T. (2005) The relationship between objective and subjective ratings of disfigurement severity, and psychological adjustment. *Body Image: An International Journal of Research*, 2: 151–9.

Moss, T. and Carr, T. (2004) Understanding adjustment to disfigurement: the role of the self-concept. *Psychology and Health*, 19: 737–48.

Mouradian, W.E. (2001) Deficits versus strengths: ethics and implications for clinical practice and research. *Cleft Palate Craniofacial Journal*, 38: 255–9.

Moyer, A. (1997) Psychological outcomes of breast-conserving surgery versus mastectomy: a meta-analytic review. *Health Psychology*, 16: 284–98.

Munro, I. (1981) The psychological effects of surgical treatment of facial deformity, in G. Lucker, K. Ribbens and J. McNamara (eds) *Psychological Aspects of Facial Form*. Ann Arbor: University of Michigan Press.

Murphy, T. and Lappe, M. (eds) (1994) *Justice and the Human Genome Project*. Berkeley: University of California Press.

Murstein, B. (1972) Physical attractiveness and marital choice. *Journal of Personality and Social Psychology*, 22: 8–12.

National Breast Implant Registry (2004) *Annual Report 2002*. Salisbury: National Breast Implant Registry.

National Burns Care Review Committee (2001) *Standards and Strategies for Burn Care: A Review of Burn Care in the British Isles*. British Association of Plastic Surgeons.

Navon, L. and Morag, A. (2003) Advanced prostate cancer patients' relationships with their spouses following hormonal therapy. *European Journal of Oncology Nursing*, 7: 73–80.

Newell, R.J. (2000a) *Body Image and Disfigurement Care*. London: Routledge.

Newell, R.J. (2000b) Psychological difficulties amongst plastic surgery ex-patients following surgery to the face: a survey. *British Journal of Plastic Surgery*, 53: 386–92.

Newell, R.J. and Clarke, M. (2000) Evaluation of a self-help leaflet in treatment of social difficulties following facial disfigurement. *International Journal of Nursing Studies*, 37: 381–8.

NHS Executive (1996) *Improving Outcomes in Breast Cancer: The Research Evidence*. London: Department of Health.

Norton, K.I., Olds, T.S., Olive, S. and Dank, S. (1996) Health concerns of artistic women gymnasts. *Sports Medicine*, 21: 321–5.

Novak, D.W. and Lerner, M.J. (1968) Rejection as a consequence of perceived similarity. *Journal of Personality and Social Psychology*, 9: 147–52.

O'Gorman, E.C. and McCrum, B. (1988) A comparison of the self-perceptions of women who have undergone mastectomy with those receiving breast reconstruction. *Irish Journal of Psychological Medicine*, 5: 26–31.

Oberle, K. and Allen, M. (1994) Breast augmentation surgery: a women's health issue. *Journal of Advanced Nursing*, 20: 844–52.

Ogden, J. (1992) *Fat Chance: The Myth of Dieting Explained*. London: Routledge.

Ogden, J. (2004) *Health Psychology*. Maidenhead: Open University Press.

Orr, D.A., Reznikoff, M. and Smith, G.M. (1989) Body image, self esteem and depression in burn-injured adolescents and young adults. *Journal of Burn Care and Rehabiltation*, 10: 454–61.

Papadopoulos, L. and Bor, R. (1999) *Psychological Approaches to Dermatology*. Leicester: BPS Books.

Papadopoulos, L., Bor, R. and Legg, C. (1999a) Coping with the disfiguring effects of vitiligo: a preliminary investigation into the effects of cognitive-behavioural therapy. *British Journal of Medical Psychology*, 72: 385–96.

Papadopoulos, L., Bor, R. and Legg, C. (1999b) Psychological factors in cutaneous disease: an overview of research. *Psychology, Health and Medicine*, 4: 107–26.

Papadopoulos, L., Bor, R., Legg, C. and Hawk, J.L.M. (1998) Impact of life events on the onset of vitiligo in adults: preliminary evidence for a psychological dimension in aetiology. *Clinical and Experimental Dermatology*, 23: 243–8.

Papadopoulos, L., Bor, R., Walker, C., Flaxman, P. and Legg, C. (2002) Different shades of meaning: illness beliefs among vitiligo sufferers. *Psychology, Health and Medicine*, 7: 425–33.

Partridge, J. (1990) *Changing Faces*. London: Penguin.

Partridge, J. (1999) Then and now: reflections on burn care past, present and future: towards a new paradigm of language and care. *Burns*, 25: 739–44.

Partridge, J. and Nash, P. (1997) The role of support groups, in R. Lansdown, N. Rumsey, E. Bradbury, T. Carr and J. Partridge (eds) *Visibly Different: Coping with Disfigurement*. Oxford: Butterworth-Heinemann.

Partridge, J. and Robinson, E. (1995) Psychological and social aspects of burns. *Burns*, 21: 453–7.

Partridge, J. and Rumsey, N. (2003) Skin scarring: new insights may make adjustment easier. *BMJ*, 326: 765.

Partridge, J., Rumsey, N. and Robinson, E. (1997) An evaluation of a pilot disfigurement support unit. Report for the Nuffield Provincial Hospital Trust.

Payne, D.K., Biggs, C., Tran, K.N., Borgen, P.I. and Massie, M.J. (2000) Women's regrets after bilateral prophylactic mastectomy. *Annals of Surgical Oncology*, 7: 150–4.

Pendley, J.S., Dahlquist, L.M. and Dreyer, Z. (1997) Body image and psychosocial adjustment in adolescent cancer survivors. *Journal of Pediatric Psychology*, 22: 29–43.

Penton-Voak, I.S. and Perrett, D.I. (2000a) Consistency and individual differences in facial attractiveness judgements – an evolutionary perspective. *Social Research*, 67: 219–44.

Penton-Voak, I.S. and Perrett, D.I. (2000b) Female preference for male faces changes cyclically – further evidence. *Evolution and Human Behaviour*, 20: 295–307.

Perrett, D.I. and Moore, F. (2004) Face Values. *New Scientist*.

Perrin, F. (1921) Physical attractiveness and repulsiveness. *Journal of Experimental Psychology*, 4: 203–17.

Pertschuk, M.J., Sarwer, D.B., Wadden, T.A. and Whitaker, L.A. (1998) Body image dissatisfaction in male cosmetic surgery patients. *Aesthetic Plastic Surgery*, 22: 20–4.

Peter, J. and Chinsky, R. (1974) Sociological aspects of cleft palate adults: 1 marriage. *Cleft Palate Journal* 11: 295–309.

Phillips, K.A. (2002) Body image and body dysmorphic disorder, in T.F. Cash and T. Pruzinsky (eds) *Body Image: A Handbook of Theory, Research and Clinical Practice*. London: The Guilford Press.

Pickering, P. (1991) Ethics and the human genome. *Bulletin of Medical Ethics*, Oct 1991, 25–31.

Piff, C. (1998) Body image: a patient's perspective. *British Journal of Theatre Nursing*, 8: 13–14.

Pillemer, F. and Cook, K. (1989) The psychosocial adjustment of pediatric craniofacial patients after surgery. *Cleft Palate and Craniofacial Journal*, 26: 207.

Pope, A.W. (1999) Points of risk and opportunity for parents of children with craniofacial conditions. *The Cleft Palate Craniofacial Journal*, 36: 36–9.

Pope, A.W. and Ward, J. (1997) Self perceived facial appearance and psychosocial adjustment in preadolescents with craniofacial anomalies. *Cleft Palate Craniofacial Journal*, 34: 396–401.

Porter, J.R., Beuf, A.H., Lerner, A. and Nordlund, J. (1986) Psychosocial effect of vitiligo: a comparison of vitiligo patients with 'normal' control subjects, with psoriasis patients, and with patients with other pigmentary disorders. *Journal of the American Academy of Dermatology*, 15: 220–4.

Porter, J.R., Beuf, A.H., Lerner, A. and Nordlund, J. (1990) The effects of vitiligo on sexual relationships. *Journal of the American Academy of Dermatology*, 22: 221–2.

Price, B. (1990) *Body Image: Nursing Concepts and Care*. Englewood Cliffs, NJ: Prentice Hall.

Price, B. (1992) Living with altered body image: the cancer experience. *British Journal of Nursing*, 1: 641–5.

Prokhorov, A., Perry, C., Kelder, S. and Kleep, K. (1993) Lifestyle values of adolescents: results from the Minnesota Heart Health Youth Program. *Adolescence*, 28: 637–47.

Pruzinsky, T. (2002) Body image adaptation to reconstructive surgery for acquired disfigurement, in T.F. Cash and T. Pruzinsky (eds) *Body Image: A Handbook of Theory, Research and Clinical Practice*, pp. 440–9. London: The Guilford Press.

Pruzinsky, T. (2004) Enhancing quality of life in medical populations: a vision for body image assessment and rehabilitation as standards of care. *Body Image*, 1: 71–81.

Pruzinsky, T. and Cash, T.F. (2002) Understanding body images: historical and contemporary perspectives, in T.F. Cash and T. Pruzinsky (eds) *Body Image: A Handbook of Theory, Research and Clinical Practice*, pp. 3–12. London: The Guilford Press.

Prynn, J. (2004) Whisper it . . . but men are joining the slimming set. *Evening Standard*, 4 November.

Radley, A. (2001) Using photography in health-related research. *Health Psychology Update*, 10: 3–5.

Ramsey, B. and O'Reagan, M. (1988) A survey of the social and psychological effects of psoriasis. *British Journal of Dermatology*, 118: 195–201.

Rapp, S., Exum, M.L., Reboussin, D.M., Feldman, S.R., Fleischer, A. and Clark, A. (1997) The physical, psychological and social impact of psoriasis. *Journal of Health Psychology*, 2: 525–37.

Reaby, L.L. (1998) The quality and coping patterns of women's decision-making regarding breast cancer surgery. *Psycho-Oncology*, 7: 252–62.

Reaby, L.L. and Hort, L.K. (1995) Postmastectomy attitudes in women who wear external breast prostheses compared to those who have undergone breast reconstruction. *Journal of Behavioural Medicine*, 18: 55–67.

Richman, L. and Millard, T. (1997) Cleft lip and palate: longitudinal behaviour and relationships to behaviour and achievement. *Journal of Paediatric Psychology*, 22: 487–94.

Rieves, L. and Cash, T.F. (1996) Social developmental factors and women's body image attitudes. *Journal of Social Behavior and Personality*, 11: 63–78.

Rizvi, S.L., Stice, E. and Agras, W.S. (1999) Natural history of disordered eating attitudes and behaviours over a 6-year period. *International Journal of Eating Disorders*, 26: 406–13.

Roberts-Harry, D. (1997) Anthropometry: the physical measurement of visible differences, in R. Lansdown, N. Rumsey, E. Bradbury, T. Carr and J. Partridge (eds) *Visibly Different: Coping with Disfigurement*. Oxford: Butterworth-Heinemann.

Robinson, E. (1997) Psychological research on visible differences in adults, in R. Lansdown, N. Rumsey, E. Bradbury, T. Carr and J. Partridge (1997) *Visibly Different: Coping with Disfigurement*. Oxford: Butterworth-Heinemann.

Robinson, E., Rumsey, N. and Partridge, J. (1996) An evaluation of the impact of social interaction skills training for facially disfigured people. *British Journal of Plastic Surgery*, 49: 281–9.

Robson, C. (2002) *Real World Research*. Oxford: Blackwell.

Rodin, J., Silberstein, L. and Streigel Moore, R. (1985) Women and weight: a normative discontent, in T. Sonderegger (ed.) *Nebraska Symposium on Motivation*, 32: *Psychology and Gender*, pp. 267–308. Lincoln: University of Nebraska Press.

Rosen, M.C., Orosan-Weine, P. and Tang, T. (1997) Critical experiences in the development of body image. *Eating Disorders: The Journal of Prevention and Treatment*, 5: 151–204.

Rosman, S. (2004) Cancer and stigma: experience of patients with chemotherapy-induced alopecia, *Patient Education and Counselling*, 52: 333–9.

Rowland, J. (1990) Developmental stage and adaptation: child and adolescent model, in J.C. Holland and J. H. Rowland (eds) *Handbook of Psycho-oncology*. Oxford: Oxford University Press.

Royal College of Surgeons of England (2003) *Facial Transplantation: Working Party Report*. London: Royal College of Surgeons of England.

Rucker, C.E. III and Cash, T.F. (1992) Body images, body-size perceptions, and eating behaviors among African-American and white college women. *International Journal of Eating Disorders*, 12: 291–9.

Rumsey, N. (1983) Psychological problems associated with facial disfigurement. Unpublished doctoral thesis, North East London Polytechnic, London.

Rumsey, N. (1997) Historical and anthropological perspectives on appearance, in R. Lansdown, N. Rumsey, E. Bradbury, T. Carr and J. Partridge (1997) *Visibly Different: Coping With Disfigurement*. Oxford: Butterworth-Heinemann.

Rumsey, N. (2002a) Optimizing body image in disfiguring congenital conditions: surgical and psychosocial interventions, in T.F. Cash and T. Pruzinksy (eds) *Body Image: A Handbook of Theory, Research and Clinical Practice*. London: The Guilford Press.

Rumsey, N. (2002b) Body image and congenital conditions with visible differences, in T.F. Cash and T. Pruzinksy (eds) *Body Image: A Handbook of Theory, Research and Clinical Practice*. London: The Guilford Press.

Rumsey, N. (2004) Psychological aspects of face transplantation: read the small print carefully. *American Journal of Bioethics*, 4: 10–13.

Rumsey, N. and Harcourt, D. (2004) Body image and disfigurement: issues and interventions. *Body Image*, 1: 83–97.

Rumsey, N., Bull, R. and Gahagan, D. (1982) The effect of facial disfigurement on the proxemic behaviour of the general public. *Journal of Applied Social Psychology*, 12: 137–50.

Rumsey, N., Bull, R. and Gahagan, D. (1986) A preliminary study of the potential social skills for improving the quality of social interaction for the facially disfigured. *Social Behaviour*, 1: 143–5.

Rumsey, N., Clarke, A. and Musa, M. (2002) Altered body image: the psychosocial needs of patients. *British Journal of Community Nursing*, 7: 563–6.

Rumsey, N., Clarke, A. and White, P. (2003a) Exploring the psychosocial concerns of outpatients with disfiguring conditions. *Journal of Wound Care*, 12: 247–52.

Rumsey, N., Clarke, A., White, P. and Hooper, E. (2003b) Investigating the appearance-related concerns of people with hand injuries. *British Journal of Hand Therapy*, 8: 57–61.

Rumsey, N., Clarke, A., White, P., Wyn-Williams, M. and Garlick, W. (2004) Altered body image: appearance-related concerns of people with visible disfigurement. *Journal of Advanced Nursing*, 48: 443–53.

Rusch, M.D., Grunert, B.K., Sanger, J.R., Dzwierzynski, W.W. and Matloub, H.S. (2000) Psychological adjustment in children after traumatic disfiguring injuries: a 12 month follow-up. *Plastic and Reconstructive Surgery*, 106: 1451–8.

Rutzen, S. (1973) The social importance of orthodontic rehabilitation: report of a 5 year follow-up study. *Journal of Health and Social Behavior*, 14: 233–40.

Sambler, G. and Hopkins, A. (1986) Being epileptic: coming to terms with stigma. *Sociology of Health and Illness*, 8: 26–43.

Santrock, J.W. (2001) *Adolescence*. New York: McGraw-Hill.

Sarwer, D.B. (2002) Cosmetic surgery and changes in body image, in T.F. Cash and T. Pruzinsky (eds) *Body Image: A Handbook of Theory, Research and Clinical Practice*. London: The Guilford Press.

Sarwer, D.B. and Crerand, C.E. (2004) Body image and cosmetic medical treatments. *Body Image*, 1: 99–111.

Sarwer, D.B., Wadden, T.A., Pertschuk, M.J. and Whitaker, L.A. (1998) The psychology of cosmetic surgery: a review and reconceptualisation. *Clinical Psychology Review*, 18: 1–22.

Sarwer, D.B., Wadden, T.A., Pertschuk, M.J. and Whitaker, L.A. (1997) Body image dissatisfaction and body dysmorphic disorder in 100 cosmetic surgery patients. *Plastic and Reconstructive Surgery*, 101: 1644–9.

Schilder, P. (1935) *The Image and Appearance of the Human Body*. New York: International Universities Press.

Schwartz, M.B. and Brownell, K.D. (2004) Obesity and body image. *Body Image*, 1: 43–56.

Searle, A., Vedhara, V., Norman, P., Frost, A. and Harrad, R. (2000) Compliance with eye patching in children and its psychosocial effects: a qualitative application of protection motivation theory. *Psychology, Health and Medicine*, 5: 43–54.

Secord, P. (1958) Facial features and interference processes in interpersonal attraction, in R. Tagiuiri and L. Petrullo (eds) *Person Perception and Interpersonal Behavior*. Stanford, CA: Stanford University Press.

Seligman, M. (1998) *Learned Optimism: How to Change Your Mind and Your Life*. New York: Pocket Books.

Shakespeare, V. and Cole, R.P. (1997) Measuring patient-based outcomes in a plastic surgery service: breast reduction surgical patients. *British Journal of Plastic Surgery*, 50: 242–8.

Shaw, W. (1981) The influence of children's dentofacial appearance on their social attractiveness as judged by peers and lay adults. *American Journal of Orthodontics*, 79: 399–415.

Sheerin, D., Macleod, M. and Kusumakar, V. (1995) Psychosocial adjustment in children with port-wine stains and prominent ears. *Journal of the American Academy of Child and Adolescent Psychiatry*, 34: 1637–47.

Shepherd, J.P. (1989) Surgical, socio-economic and forensic aspects of assault: a review. *British Journal of Oral and Maxillofacial Surgery*, 27: 89–98.

Sigall, H. and Aronson, E. (1969) Liking for an evaluator as a function of her physical attractiveness and nature of the evaluation. *Journal of Experimental Social Psychology*, 5: 93–100.

Smith, P. (1999) *The nature of school bullying: A cross national perspective.* London: Routledge.

Smolak, L. (2004) Body image in children and adolescents: where do we go from here? *Body Image*, 1: 15–28.

Smolak, L., Levine, M.P. and Schermer, F. (1998) A controlled evaluation of an elementary primary school prevention program for eating problems. *Journal of Psychosomatic Research*, 44: 339–54.

Smolak, L., Levine, M.P. and Schermer, F. (1999) Parental input and weight concerns among elementary school children. *International Journal of Eating Disorders*, 25: 263–71.

Somerfield, M. (1997) The utility of systems models of stress and coping for applied research: the case of cancer adaptation. *Journal of Health Psychology*, 2: 133–51.

Speltz, M., Goodell, E., Endriga, M. and Clarren, S. (1994) Feeding interactions of infants with unrepaired cleft lip and/or palate. *Infant Behavior Development*, 17: 131–40.

Speltz, M., Norton, K., Goodell, E. and Clarren, S. (1993) Psychological functioning of children with craniofacial anomalies and their mothers: follow up from late infancy to school-entry. *Cleft Palate Journal*, 30: 482–9.

Spicer, J. (2002) Appearance-related concern in older adults with skin disorder: an exploratory study. Unpublished doctoral thesis, Exeter University.

Spira, M., Chizen, J., Gerow, F. and Hardy, S. (1966) Plastic surgery in the Texas prison system. *British Journal of Plastic Surgery*, 19: 364–71.

Stanford, J.N. and McCabe, M.P. (2002) Body image ideal among males and females: sociocultural influences and focus on different body parts. *Journal of Health Psychology*, 7: 675–84.

Starr, P. (1980) Facial attractiveness and behavior of patients with cleft lip and/or palate. *Psychological Reports*, 46: 579–82.

Stephan, C. and Langois, J. (1984) Baby beautiful: adult attributions of infant competence as a function of infant attractiveness. *Child Development*, 55: 576–85.

Stormer, S.M. and Thompson, J.K. (1996) Explanations of body image disturbance: a test of maturational status, negative verbal commentary, social comparison and sociocultural hypotheses. *International Journal of Eating Disorders*, 19: 193–202.

Strauss, R.P. (1985) Culture, rehabilitation and facial birth defects: international case studies. *Cleft Palate Journal*, 21: 56–62.

Strauss, R.P. (2001) 'Only skin deep': health, resilience and craniofacial care. *Cleft Palate Craniofacial Journal*, 38: 226–30.

Strauss, R.P. and Broder, H. (1991) Directions and issues in psychosocial research and methods as applied to cleft lip and palate and craniofacial anomalies. *Cleft Palate Craniofacial Journal*, 28: 150–6.

Strenta, A. and Kleck, R. (1985) Physical disability and the attribution dilemma: perceiving the causes of social behavior. *Journal of Social and Clinical Psychology*, 3: 129–42.

Sund, B. (2000) *New Developments in Wound Care*. London: PJB Publications.

Tanner, J.L., Dechert, M.P. and Frieden, I.J. (1998) Growing up with a facial hemangioma: parent and child coping and adaptation. *Pediatrics*, 101: 446–52.

Tantleff-Dunn, S. and Thompson, J.K. (1998) Body image and appearance-related feedback: recall, judgement and affective response. *Journal of Social and Clinical Psychology*, 17: 319–40.

Tashakkori, A. and Teddlie, C. (1998) *Mixed Methodology: Combining Qualitative and Quantitative Approaches*. London: SAGE Publications.

Thomas, C.M., Keery, H., Williams, R. and Thompson, J.K. (1998) The fear of appearance evaluation scale: development and preliminary validation. Paper presented at the Association for the Advancement of Behavior Therapy, Washington, DC.

Thompson, A.R. and Kent, G. (2001) Adjusting to disfigurement: processes involved in dealing with being visibly different. *Clinical Psychology Review*, 21: 663–82.

Thompson, A.R., Kent, G. and Smith, J.A. (2002) Living with vitiligo: dealing with difference. *British Journal of Health Psychology*, 7: 213–25.

Thompson, J.K. (1990) *Body Image and Disturbance*. Oxford: Pergamon Press.

Thompson, J.K. (2004) The (mis)measurement of body image: ten strategies to improve assessment for applied and research purposes. *Body Image*, 1: 7–14.

Thompson, J.K. and Van den Berg, P. (2002) Measuring body image attitudes among adolescents and adults, in T.F. Cash and T. Pruzinsky (eds) *Body Image: A Handbook of Theory, Research and Clinical Practice*. London: The Guilford Press.

Thompson, J.K., Heinberg, L.J., Altabe, M. and Tantleff-Dunn, S. (1999) *Exacting Beauty: Theory, Assessment and Treatment of Body Image Disturbance*. Washington, DC: APA.

Tiggemann, M. (2002) Media influences on body image development, in T.F. Cash and T. Pruzinsky (eds) *Body Image: A Handbook of Theory, Research and Clinical Practice*, pp. 91–8. London: The Guilford Press.

Tiggemann, M. (2004) Body image across the adult lifespan: stability and change. *Body Image*, 1: 29–41.

Tiggemann, M. and Pennington, B. (1990) The development of gender differences in body-size dissatisfaction. *Australian Psychologist*, 25: 301–11.

Tobiasen, J.M. and Hiebert, J.M. (1993) Clefting and psychosocial adjustment. *Clinical Plastic Surgery*, 20: 623–31.

Trust, D. (1977) Skin Deep: An Introduction to Skin Camouflage and Disfigurement Therapy. Edinburgh: Harris.

Tunalcy, J.R., Walsh, S. and Nicholson, P. (1999) 'I'm not bad for my age': the meaning of body size and eating in the lives of older women. *Ageing and Society*, 19: 741–59.

Turner, S., Thomas, P., Dowell, T., Rumsey, N. and Sandy, J. (1997) Psychological outcomes amongst cleft patients and their families. *British Journal of Plastic Surgery*, 50: 1–10.

Udry, J. (1965) Structural correlates of feminine beauty preferences in Britain and the U.S.: a comparison. *Sociology and Social Research*, 49: 330–42.

Udry, J. and Eckland, B. (1984) Benefits of being attractive: differential payoffs for men and women. *Psychological Reports*, 54: 47–56.

Vamos, M. (1990) Body image in rheumatoid arthritis: the relevance of hand appearance to desire for surgery. *British Journal of Medical Psychology*, 63: 267–77.

Van der Donk, J., Hunfield, J., Passcher, J., Knegt-Junk, K. and Nieboer, C. (1994) Quality of life and maladjustment associated with hair loss in women with alopecia androgenetic. *Social Science and Medicine*, 38: 159–63.

Vance, Y., Morse, R.C., Jenney, M.E. and Eiser, C. (2001) Issues in measuring quality of life in childhood cancer: measures, proxies, and parental mental health. *Journal of Childhood Psychology and Psychiatry*, 42: 661–7.

Veale, D. (2004) Advances in a cognitive behavioural model of body dysmorphic disorder. *Body Image*, 1: 113–25.

Vincent, M. and McCabe, M. (2000) Gender differences among adolescents in family and peer influences on body dissatisfaction, weight loss, and binge eating behaviors. *Journal of Youth and Adolescence*, 29: 205–21.

Wahl, A.K., Gjengedal, E. and Hanestad, B.R. (2002) The bodily suffering of living with severe psoriasis: in-depth interviews with 22 hospitalized patients with psoriasis. *Qualitative Health Research*, 12: 250–61.

Walden, K.J., Thompson, J.K. and Wells, K.E. (1997) Body image and psychological sequelae of silicone breast explantation: preliminary findings. *Plastic and Reconstructive Surgery*, 100: 1299–306.

Wallace, L.M. and Lees, J. (1988) A psychological follow-up study of adult patients discharged from a British burn unit. *Burns*, 14: 39–45.

Wallace, M. (2004) The appearance-related concerns of adolescents who have undergone treatment for cancer. Paper presented at the British Psychological Society Division of Health Psychology Annual Conference, Edinburgh, September 2004.

Walters, E. (1997) Problems faced by children and families living with visible differences, in R. Lansdown, N. Rumsey, E. Bradbury, T. Carr and J. Partridge (eds) *Visibly Different: Coping With Disfigurement*. Oxford: Butterworth-Heinemann.

Walster, E., Aronson, E., Abrahams, D. and Rottman, L. (1966) The importance of physical attractiveness in dating behavior. *Journal of Personality and Social Psychology*, 4: 508–16.

Ward, C. (1999) The technological imperative in the treatment of craniofacial deformity. *Cleft Palate Craniofacial Journal*, 36: 1–2.

Wardle, J. and Collins, E. (1998) Body dissatisfaction: Social and emotional influences in adolescent girls. Unpublished manuscript, University College, London.

Wardle, J. and Marsland, L. (1990) Adolescent concerns about weight and eating: a social-developmental perspective. *Journal of Psychosomatic Research*, 34: 377–91.

Warnock, M. (1992) Ethical challenges of embryo manipulation. *British Medical Journal*, 304: 1045–9.

White, C.A. (2000) Body image dimensions and cancer: a heuristic cognitive behavioural model. *Psycho-Oncology*, 9: 183–92.

White, C.A. (2002) Body image issues in oncology, in T.F. Cash and T. Pruzinsky (eds) *Body Image: A Handbook of Theory, Research and Clinical Practice.* London: The Guilford Press.

Wilcox, S. (1997) Age and gender in relation to body attitudes: is there a double standard of ageing? *Psychology of Women Quarterly,* 21: 549–65.

Williams, J., Wood, C. and Cunningham-Warburton, P. (1999) A narrative study of chemotherapy-induced alopecia. *Oncology Nursing Forum,* 26: 1463–8.

Wood, K.C., Becker, J.A. and Thompson, J.K. (1998) The commentary interpretation scale: a measure of judgment of neutral appearance commentary. Unpublished manuscript, University of South Florida.

Wright, S.R. (2002) Appearance, disfigurement and self-perceptions. Unpublished MSc dissertation, University of the West of England, Bristol.

Yardley, L. (2001) Mixing theories: (how) can qualitative and quantitative health psychology research be combined? *Health Psychology Update,* 10: 6–9.

YouGov (2003) *Opinion Poll for the Charity Changing Faces,* Changing Faces, London.

Young, V.L., Nemecek, J.R. and Nemecek, D.A. (1994) The efficacy of breast augmentation: breast size increase, patient satisfaction and psychological effects. *Plastic and Reconstructive Surgery,* 94: 958–69.

Zabora, J., Brintzenhofeszoc, K., Curbow, B., Hooker, C. and Piantadosi, S. (2001) the prevalence of psychologial distress by cancer site. *Psycho-Oncology* 10: 19–28.

Ziegelmann, J.P., Griva, K., Hankins, M., Davenport, A., Thompson, D. and Newman, S. (2002) The Transplant Effects Questionnaire (TxEQ): the development of a questionnaire for assessing the multidimensional outcome of organ transplantation – example of end stage renal disease (ERSD). *British Journal of Health Psychology,* 7: 393–408.

Zigmond, A.S. and Snaith, R.P. (1983) The Hospital Anxiety and Depression Scale. *Acta Psychiatrica Scandinavica,* 67: 361–70.

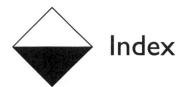

# Index

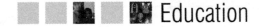
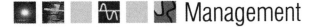
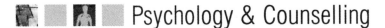
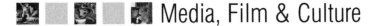
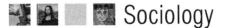
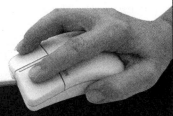
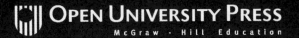